The Truth About Depression and How Women
Can Heal Their Bodies to Reclaim Their Lives

A Mind
of Your
Own

KELLY BROGAN, MD
with Kristin Loberg

Thorsons

This book contains advice and information relating to health care. It is not intended to replace medical advice and should be used to supplement rather than replace regular care by your doctor. It is recommended that you seek medical advice before embarking on any medical programme or treatment. All efforts have been made to assure the accuracy of the information contained in this book as of the date of publication. The publisher and the author disclaim liability for any medical outcomes that may occur as a result of applying the methods suggested in this book.

Thorsons
An imprint of HarperCollins*Publishers*
1 London Bridge Street
London SE1 9GF

www.harpercollins.co.uk

First published in the US by Harper Wave, an imprint of HarperCollins*Publishers* 2016
This UK edition published by Thorsons 2016

13

Text © Kelly Brogan 2016

Kelly Brogan asserts the moral right to be
identified as the author of this work

A catalogue record of this book is
available from the British Library

ISBN 978-0-00-812800-5

Printed and bound by CPI Group (UK) Ltd, Croydon, CR0 4YY

MIX
Paper from
responsible sources
FSC www.fsc.org **FSC™ C007454**

FSC™ is a non-profit international organisation established to promote
the responsible management of the world's forests. Products carrying the
FSC label are independently certified to assure consumers that they come
from forests that are managed to meet the social, economic and
ecological needs of present and future generations,
and other controlled sources.

Find out more about HarperCollins and the environment at
www.harpercollins.co.uk/green

To the legacy of Dr. Nicholas Gonzalez
and to all of the light workers
who illuminate the path for my daughters,
and everyone's daughters.

Contents

A Mind of Your Own

Psych—It's Not All in Your Head

All along the history of medicine, the really great physicians were peculiarly free from the bondage of drugs.
—SIR WILLIAM OSLER (1849–1919)

If you've picked up this book, then chances are you can relate to any of the following: persistent distress, malaise, anxiety, inner agitation, fatigue, low libido, poor memory, irritability, insomnia, sense of hopelessness, and feeling overwhelmed and trapped but emotionally flat. You might wake up most mornings unmotivated and uninspired, and you drag yourself around all day waiting for it to end (or waiting for a drink). Maybe you feel a sense of dread or panic without knowing why. You can't silence the negative thoughts, which puts you on edge. Sometimes it seems like you could let loose an endless stream of tears, or perhaps you can't remember the last time you cared enough about something to cry. All of these descriptions are symptoms that typically fall under a diagnosis of clinical depression. And if you were to seek help through conventional medicine, even if you don't consider yourself "depressed," you'd likely be handed a prescription for an antidepressant, joining the more than 30 million users in America. You might already be part of this community and feel like your fate is now sealed.

It doesn't have to be.

Over the past twenty-five years, ever since the FDA approval of Prozac-type medications, we've been taught that drugs can improve the symptoms of or even cure mental illness, particularly depression and anxiety disorders. Today they are among the most prescribed, best-selling drugs.[1] This has led to one of the most silent and underestimated tragedies in the history of modern health care.

I am a practicing psychiatrist with a degree in cognitive neuroscience from MIT, an MD from Weill Cornell Medical College, and clinical training from NYU School of Medicine, and I care deeply for women struggling with their well-being. I'm compelled to share what I've learned from witnessing the corruption of modern psychiatry and its sordid history while investigating holistic methods that focus on nutrition, meditation, and physical activity—what some practitioners are calling lifestyle medicine because the approach involves changes in everyday *lifestyle* habits, not the use of pharmaceuticals. While such drug-free methods are entirely evidence-based, they are virtually unknown in this age of the quick fix.

Let's get a few facts straight from the get-go. I'm not a conspiracy theorist. I'm not even that politically minded, but I do like to think for myself. I'm a natural skeptic and pragmatist. These days, there are a couple of issues in my line of work that are making my blood boil, and I'm working to connect the dots between them to help establish a framework for a truth in science "sniff-test." For one, symptoms of mental illness are not entirely a psychological problem, nor are they purely a neurochemical issue (and, as we'll see shortly, *not a single study* has proven that depression is caused by a chemical imbalance in the brain). Depression is merely a symptom, a sign that something is off balance or ill in the body that needs to be remedied.

And two, depression is a grossly misdiagnosed and mistreated condition today, especially among women—one in seven of whom is being medicated. (For reasons we'll be exploring, women experience more than *twice* the rate of depression as men, regardless of race or ethnic background. One in four women in their forties and fifties use psychiatric drugs.)[2] Although I was trained to think that antidepressants are to the depressed (and to the anxious, panicked, OCD, IBS, PTSD, bulimic, anorexic, and so on) what eyeglasses are to the poor-sighted, I no longer buy into this bill of goods. And after reading this book, you too may think twice about all you thought you understood about the causes of depression.

We owe most of our mental illnesses—including their kissing cousins such as chronic worry, fogginess, and crankiness—to lifestyle factors and undiagnosed physiological conditions that develop in places far from the brain, such as the gut and thyroid. That's right: you might owe your gloominess and unremitting unease to an imbalance that is only indirectly related to your brain's internal chemistry. Indeed, what you eat for breakfast (think whole wheat toast, fresh OJ, milk, and multigrain cereal) and how you deal with that high cholesterol and afternoon headache (think Lipitor and Advil) could have everything to do with the causes and symptoms of your depression. And if you think a chemical pill can save, cure, or "correct" you, you're dead wrong. That is about as misguided as taking aspirin for a nail stuck in your foot.

While it's well documented that multiple forces—such as a tragic life event or the fallout from hormonal shifts—can trigger symptoms labeled (and treated) as depression, no one has explained the potential for antidepressants to irreversibly disable the body's natural healing mechanisms. Despite what you've been led to believe, antidepressants have repeatedly been shown in long-term scientific studies to *worsen* the course of mental illness—to say nothing of the risks of liver damage, abnormal bleeding, weight gain, sexual dysfunction, and reduced cognitive function that they entail. The dirtiest little secret of all is the fact that antidepressants are among the most difficult drugs to taper from, more so than alcohol and opiates. While you might call it "going through withdrawal," we medical professionals have been instructed by Big Pharma to call it "discontinuation syndrome," which is characterized by fiercely debilitating physical and psychological reactions.

So unlike most psychiatrists, I'm not one to diagnose a "permanent" condition, write a prescription, and send my patient on her merry way—the knee-jerk gold standard in my field today. Nor do I have her sit on a couch and talk about her problems endlessly. Much to the contrary, my first item of business is to discuss her medical and personal history, including questions that give me a sense of her life's exposures since birth, from noxious chemical encounters to whether or not she was born through the birth canal and breast-fed. I also order lab tests that help me take in the bigger picture of her total biology; these are noninvasive screenings that most psychiatrists and general practitioners don't even think about doing (and in this book you'll be learning about these easy-to-obtain tests as tools to help you personalize your path to healing).

While I acknowledge my patient's past experiences, I also focus on what's unfolding today from a cellular standpoint and the potential impairment ("dysregulation") of her immune system. The medical literature has emphasized the role of inflammation in mental illness for more than twenty years. I listen closely and ask her about her current lifestyle, a dismissed and neglected variable in conventional medicine. I reflect on her entirety, considering factors like how much sugar she consumes and other dietary habits, how well her gut and its microbial communities are collaborating, hormone levels such as thyroid and cortisol, genetic variants in her DNA that can put her at a higher risk for symptoms of depression, her beliefs about health, and her intentions for our work together. (And, yes, this takes hours.)

All of my patients share similar goals: they want to feel physically vibrant and emotionally balanced, which I believe is everyone's birthright—not perpetually drained, unsettled, mentally foggy, and unable to enjoy life. Under my guidance, they achieve these goals through very simple and straightforward strategies: dietary modifications (more healthy fats and less sugar, dairy, and gluten); natural supplements like B vitamins and probiotics that don't require a prescription and can even be delivered through certain foods; minimizing exposures to biology-disrupting toxicants*

---

* A toxicant refers to any toxic substance, though it's often a term used to indicate substances made by humans or introduced into the environment by human activity. The term *toxin*, on the other hand, refers to toxicants produced naturally by a living organism.

like fluoride in tap water and fragrances in cosmetics; harnessing the power of sufficient sleep and physical movement; and practicing behavioral techniques aimed at promoting the relaxation response. These basic lifestyle interventions facilitate the body's powerful self-healing mechanisms, and there's plenty of science to support these protocols. This isn't New Age medicine; I will prove my claims and back my recommendations with current peer-reviewed studies from the world's most esteemed publications.

I do not deny that I have developed a sometimes belligerent relationship with much of conventional medicine over the past several years. After having witnessed the devastation this paradigm has wrought upon the lives of hundreds of my patients, I'm convinced that the pharmaceutical industry and its bedfellows, concealed behind official titles such as certain medical societies and associations, have created an illusion of science where none exists, in the service of profit over professional responsibility. I will myth bust just about everything you think you know about the role of drugs in the treatment of depression and anxiety. It's time to turn the lights on in this dark room. Let's open up this conversation and embrace a perspective on depression that radically challenges mainstream assumptions and theories. If I do my job well, you'll never look at another ad for an antidepressant again in quite the same way.

Admittedly, I haven't always been militant about my now unshakable, passionate belief in the effectiveness of holistic, drug-free medicine to heal women's minds, moods, and memory. I've crossed over from the other side in many ways, having once been a dyed-in-the-wool allopathic doctor. I'm from a family that regards conventional medicine as a guiding light. I was always interested in neuroscience and the promise of understanding behavior and pathology, and I pursued psychiatry for that reason. My inner feminist wasn't totally satisfied, however, until I began to specialize in women's health. There's a growing field in psychiatry called perinatal or reproductive psychiatry that focuses on the risk-benefit analysis of treating women during their reproductive years. This is a uniquely vulnerable time period, particularly if a woman is contemplating taking drugs while simultaneously planning a pregnancy or is already pregnant. I soon began to feel constrained by the medication and/or talk therapy model of treating depression, and I delved into how to cultivate better options for not just women in their reproductive years but all women across the entire life cycle.

The further I stepped away from traditional psychiatry, the more I started to ask questions few others in my field were raising, principally "Why?" Why have the body and mind become dysfunctional in so many millions of women? Are we inherently broken? Why have we gotten so much sicker in the past century when our DNA—the same DNA we've had for millions of years—hasn't changed? Or are doctors just getting better at labeling symptoms under the wastebasket diagnosis that is depression?

These are among the many questions addressed in this book; the answers pave the way to a revolutionary—and by that I mean extremely self-empowering!—new approach to well-being.

I've seen extraordinary turnarounds in health. Take, for instance, the fifty-six-year-old woman who entered my office complaining of low energy, pervasive pain, dry skin, constipation, weight gain, and forgetfulness. She was taking an antidepressant and a cholesterol-lowering statin but feeling progressively worse and desperate for answers. Within months, she was off all meds, her cholesterol level optimized, and her "depression" vanished. Or consider the thirty-two-year-old woman with a history of premenstrual syndrome (PMS) for which she'd taken birth control pills until trying to become pregnant. When she came in to see me, she was on an antidepressant for her flat mood and fatigue and was unable to conceive despite two years of trying. What followed next was not a miracle but rather something I witness every day in my practice. With a few easy changes to her diet and a combination of other lifestyle strategies—the same ones outlined in this book—she was soon prescription-free and pregnant. She also was symptom-free for the first time in her life.

You'll be meeting many women in this book whose stories speak for themselves and are emblematic of millions of others who live with unnecessary, life-depleting depression. And I trust that you'll relate to one or more of them. Whether you're currently taking antidepressants or not, this book has something for every woman who struggles to feel like the radiant self she deserves to be. I see a lot of patients who have "tried everything" and have been to the country's top doctors. In fact, a good percentage of my practice involves treating *other physicians and psychiatrists.*

Many women credit me with the initiation of life transformation. Because I believe passionately in the power of lifestyle medicine to produce changes that are greater than the sum of their parts—bigger, bolder shifts in how we relate to life, spirituality, the environment, and even authorities—I see myself as an ambassador to a new way of experiencing health and well-being. This way of being may be built on the ashes of suffering, but may be the way to rise up, phoenix-like, emboldened, and stronger than ever. That strength and resilience is yours, and it follows you everywhere you take it.

I've divided the book into two parts. Part 1: "The Truth About Depression," takes you on a tour of your mental health's friends and enemies, from everyday foods to common prescription and over-the-counter medications. You'll soon be consuming *more* saturated fat and cholesterol and shopping differently in the grocery store and drugstore. In compelling detail, backed by science, I'll expose the stunning relationship between your gut's health and mental health. And I'll do so within the context of inflammation, an overused buzzword today that most people still don't truly comprehend, especially when it comes to its critical role in depression. I will prove that depression is often a result of chronic inflammation—simple as that. I also will explain the underlying responsibilities of your immune system in orchestrating all matters of mental health.

Part 1 includes an overview of the latest research on how we can dramatically alter our genetic destiny—how our genes express themselves, including those directly related to mood—through the everyday choices we make in food and activities. The goal of Part 1 is to prep you for the program you'll embark on in Part 2: "Natural

Treatments for Whole-Body Wellness." This is where I guide you through my program, a program designed both for women not taking medications and those who are and perhaps are dreaming of tapering off. Included is a four-week plan of action, complete with menu plans and strategies for incorporating new lifestyle habits into your day.

For support and ongoing updates, you can go to my website, www.kellybroganmd.com. There you'll be able to read my blog, watch my instructional videos, access the latest scientific studies, and download materials that will help you tailor the information in this book to your personal preferences.

Once you apply to your life what you learn in these pages, you will reap more than the reward of mental stability. My patients often list the following "side benefits" to my program: feeling in control of their lives and bodies (including effortless weight management); clarity of mind and spirit; enhanced energy; and an unwavering tolerance for distress. Who wouldn't want these results? The time has come for you to have a mind of your own.

Let's get started.

PART ONE

THE TRUTH ABOUT DEPRESSION

CHAPTER 1

Decoding Depression

It's Not a Disease: What You Don't Know About
This Syndrome and How It Manifests

Depression can result from bodily imbalance rather than brain chemical imbalance.

———

The medicalization of distress obliterates meaning and creates profit.

When I talk about medicine and mental health to large audiences, I often start with the following imagery and facts: think of a woman you know who is radiantly healthy. I bet your intuition tells you she sleeps and eats well, finds purpose in her life, is active and fit, and finds time to relax and enjoy the company of others. I doubt you envision her waking up to prescription bottles, buoying her way through the day with caffeine and sugar, feeling anxious and isolated, and drinking herself to sleep at night. All of us have an intuitive sense of what health is, but many of us have lost the roadmap to optimal health, especially the kind of health that springs forth when we simply clear a path for it. The fact that one in four American women in the prime of their life is dispensed medication for a mental health condition represents a national crisis.[1]

Humans have used mind-altering substances to try to dull and deaden pain, misery, sorrow, and suffering since time immemorial, but only in the last few decades have people been persuaded that depression is a disease and that chemical antidepressants are the remedy. This is far from the truth. Many of my patients have been to multiple doctors, bumping up against the hard ceiling of what conventional medicine has to offer. Some have even tried integrative medicine, which aims to combine both traditional medicine (i.e., prescriptions) with alternative treatments (e.g., acupuncture). After all, they are told that there are great natural complements to all the wonders pharmaceutical products have to offer. But the reason they can't find a solution is because nobody has asked *why*. Why are they unwell? Why are their bodies creating symptoms that manifest as depression? Why didn't they stop to ask this important and obvious question the first time they experienced a flat mood, anxiety, insomnia, and chronic exhaustion?

Before I even get to the answers, let me be the first to tell you that the only path to a real solution is to leave the medical world you know behind. This, the journey I will take you on, is not just about symptom suppression, it's about health freedom. First let me tell you that I was once a typical doctor, not to mention a typical American who loved pizza, soda, birth control, and ibuprofen. My message is from a personal journey and thousands of hours of research that has compelled me to share the truth about prescription-based care: we've been duped.

Yes, my entire training was based on a model of disease care that offers patients only one tool—a drug—and never a shot at true wellness. We've handed over our health to those who seek to profit from it, and we've been buying into a paradigm based on the following notions:

- ▶ We are broken.
- ▶ Fear is an appropriate response to symptoms.
- ▶ We need chemicals to feel better.
- ▶ Doctors know what they are doing.
- ▶ The body is a machine requiring calibration (via drugs). A little too much of this, too little of that.

I call this collective set of notions the Western Medical Illusion. It sets up a vicious system that ushers you into lifelong customer status, dependent and disempowered.

As you can likely guess by now, I love to rant. But I do so with the best evidence science can offer, and there's a lot we know today about the real root causes of depression—and how to treat the condition safely and successfully—without a prescription pad. If there's one lesson I will drive home, it's this: shed the fear, take back your inner compass, and embrace a commitment to your best self, medication free. Even if you don't already take a prescription drug, I bet you still doubt living the rest of your life prescription free and reliant on your own inner intuition to know what's best for you. The idea of supporting your body's innate wisdom may sound quaint at best, or like dangerous hippie woo-woo at worst. From now on, I want you to embrace these new ideas:

▶ Prevention is possible.
▶ Medication treatment comes at a steep cost.
▶ Optimal health is not possible through medication.
▶ Your health is under your control.
▶ Working with lifestyle medicine—simple everyday habits that don't entail drugs—is a safe and effective way to send the body a signal of safety.

How can I make these statements, and what do I mean by life-style medicine? You're going to find out in this book, and I'll be presenting the scientific proof to answer questions you may have and to satisfy the doubtful. When I meet a woman and her family, I speak about how to reverse her anxiety, depression, mania, and even psychosis. We map out the timeline that brought her where she is and identify triggers that often fall under one or more of the following categories: food intolerances or sensitivities, blood sugar imbalances, chemical exposures, thyroid dysfunction, and nutrient deficiency. I forge a partnership with my patient and witness dramatic symptom relief within thirty days. I do this by teaching my patients how they can make simple shifts in their daily habits, starting with the diet. They increase nutrient density, eliminate inflammatory foods, balance blood sugar, and bring themselves closer to food in its ancestral state. It's the most powerful way to move the needle, because food is not just fuel. It is *information* (literally: "it puts the *form into* your body"), and its potential for healing is a wonder to me, every single day.

Achieving radical wellness takes sending the body the right information and protecting it from aggressive assault. This isn't just about mental health; it's about how mental health is a manifestation of all that your body is experiencing and your mind's interpretation of its own safety and power. It's also about how symptoms are just the visible rough edges of a gigantic submerged iceberg.

Note that none of these concepts connects with substances in the brain that might be "low." If you had to define depression right now, before reading further, chances are you'd say something about it being a "mood disorder" or "mental illness" triggered by a chemical imbalance in the brain that probably needs to be fixed through a medication like Prozac or Zoloft that will lift levels of brain chemicals associated with a good mood. But you would be mistaken.

So many patients today who are being shepherded into the psychiatric medication mill are overdiagnosed, misdiagnosed, or mistreated. Indeed, they have "brain fog," changes in metabolism, insomnia, agitation, and anxiety, but for reasons only loosely related to their brain chemicals. They have all the symptoms that are mentioned in a Cymbalta advertisement that tells them to talk to their doctor to see if Cymbalta is right for them. But it's like putting a bandage over a splinter in the skin that continues to stir inflammation and pain. It's absolutely missing an opportunity to remove the splinter and resolve the problem from the source. And it's an iconic example of how conventional medicine can make grave mistakes, something the pharmaceutical industry is more than happy to encourage.

In holistic medicine, there are no specialties. It's all connected.

Here's a classic case in point: Eva had been taking an antidepressant for two years but wanted to get off it because she was planning to get pregnant. Her doctor advised her not to stop taking the drug, which motivated her to see me. Eva explained that her saga had begun with PMS, featuring a week each month when she was irritable and prone to crying fits. Her doctor prescribed a birth control pill (a common treatment) and soon Eva was feeling even worse, with insomnia, fatigue, low libido, and a generally flat mood dogging her all month long. That's when the doctor added the Wellbutrin to "pick her up," as he said, and handle her presumed depression. From Eva's perspective, she felt that the antidepressant helped her energy level, but it had limited benefits in terms of her mood and libido. And if she took it after midnight, her insomnia was exacerbated. She soon became accustomed to feeling stable but suboptimal, and she was convinced that the medication was keeping her afloat.

The good news for Eva was that with careful preparation, she could leave medication behind—and restore her energy, her equilibrium, and her sense of control over her emotions. Step one consisted of some basic diet and exercise changes along with better stress response strategies. Step two involved stopping birth control pills and then testing her hormone levels. Just before her period, she had low cortisol and progesterone, which were likely the cause of the PMS that started her whole problem. Further testing revealed borderline low thyroid function, which may well have been the result of the contraceptives—and the cause of her increased depressive symptoms.

When Eva was ready to begin tapering off her medication, she did so following my protocol. Even as her brain and body adjusted to not having the antidepressant surging through her system anymore, her energy levels improved, her sleep problems resolved, and her anxiety lifted. Within a year she was healthy, no longer taking any prescriptions, feeling good—and pregnant.

I require my patients and I implore you to think differently about health-care decisions and consumerism. Part of my motivation in writing this book was to help you develop a new watching, questioning eye that you can bring to every experience. For my patients to be well, I know they will need to approach their health with an extreme commitment to the integrity of their mind and body. Personally, I have no intention of ever returning to a lifestyle that involves pharmaceutical products of any kind, under any circumstances.

Why?

Because we are looking at the body as an intricately woven spiderweb—when you yank one area of it, the whole thing moves. And because there is a more powerful way to heal.

It's so simple that it could be considered an act of rebellion.

You might think of yourself as averse to conflict—someone who wants to keep the peace, keep your head low, and do what's recommended. To be healthy in today's world, however, you need to access and cultivate a *reliance* on yourself. And you're going to do that by first shifting your perspective forever. Look behind the curtain and understand that medicine is not what you think it is. Drug-based medicine makes you sick. I will go so far as to say that hospital care makes you sick; though estimates vary, it's reasonable to say that hospital care claims tens if not hundreds of thousands of lives annually due to preventable medical mistakes such as wrong diagnoses and medications or surgical errors, infections, and simply screwing up an IV.[2] The Cochrane Collaboration, a London-based network of more than 31,000 researchers from more than 130 countries, conducts the world's most thorough independent analysis of health-care research. Based on data from the *British Medical Journal,* the *Journal of the American Medical Association,* and the Centers for Disease Control, it has found that prescription drugs are the third leading cause of death after heart disease and cancer.[3] And when it comes to psychotropic drugs, the Cochrane Collaboration's conclusions are compellingly uncomfortable. In the words of the Collaboration's founder, Dr. Peter Gotzsche, "Our citizens would be far better off if we removed all the psychotropic drugs from the market, as doctors are unable to handle them. It is inescapable that their availability creates more harm than good."[4]

By and large, doctors are not bad people. They are smart individuals who work hard, investing money, blood, sweat, and tears into their training. But where do doctors get their information? Whom are they told to trust? Have you ever wondered who's pulling the strings? Some of us in the medical community are beginning to speak up and to expose the fact that our training and education is, for the most part, bought.

"Unfortunately in the balance between benefits and risks, it is an uncomfortable truth that most drugs do not work in most patients."[5] Before I read this quote in the prestigious *British Medical Journal* in 2013, I had already begun to explore the evidence that there really isn't much to support the efficacy of most medications and medical interventions, particularly in psychiatry, where suppressed data and industry-funded and ghostwritten papers hide the truth. Another 2013 study published in the equally respected *Mayo Clinic Proceedings* confirmed that a whopping 40 percent of current medical practice should be thrown out.[6] Unfortunately, it takes an average of seventeen years for the data that exposes inefficacy and/or a signal of harm to trickle down into your doctor's daily routine, a time lag problem that makes medicine's standard of care evidence-based only in theory and not practice.[7] Dr. Richard Horton, the editor in chief of the much-revered *Lancet* at this writing, has broken rank and come forward about what he really thinks about published research—that it's unreliable at best, if not completely false. In a 2015 published statement, he wrote: "The case against science is straightforward: much of the scientific literature, perhaps half, may simply be untrue. Afflicted by studies with small sample sizes, tiny effects, invalid exploratory analyses, and flagrant conflicts of interest, together with an obsession for pursuing fashionable trends of dubious importance, science has taken a turn towards darkness."[8]

In 2011 the *British Medical Journal* performed a general analysis of some 2,500 common medical treatments. The goal was to determine which ones are supported by sufficient reliable evidence.[9] The results:

- ▶ 13 percent were found to be beneficial
- ▶ 23 percent were likely to be beneficial
- ▶ 8 percent were as likely to be harmful as beneficial
- ▶ 6 percent were unlikely to be beneficial
- ▶ 4 percent were likely to be harmful or ineffective

The treatments in the remaining 46 percent, the largest category, were found to be unknown in their effectiveness. Put simply, when you visit a doctor or hospital, you have only a 36 percent chance that you'll receive a treatment that has been scientifically proven to be either beneficial or likely to be beneficial. Such results are strikingly similar to those of Dr. Brian Berman, who analyzed completed Cochrane reviews of conventional medical practices, finding that 38 percent of treatments were positive and 62 percent were negative or showed "no evidence of effect."[10]

Are there exceptions? I would like to argue that there aren't. This is because the whole pharmaceutical approach is predicated on wrong-headed information. Pharmaceutical products as we know them have not been developed or studied with modern science's most relevant principles in mind, such as the complexity and power of the human microbiome, the impact of low-dose toxic exposures, autoimmune disorders as a sign of environmental overstimulation, and the fundamental importance of individual biochemistry. Because medicine operates under the now antiquated one gene, one illness, one pill rubric, efficacy will be measured through a skewed lens, and safety cannot be accurately assessed or discussed with individual patients.

Many of us move through life with a sneaking fear that the other health shoe could drop at any moment. We can easily fall prey to the belief that our breasts are ticking time bombs, that infections are just a cough or handshake away, and that life is a process of adding more medications and drugs to put out small fires as we age. Before

I stopped prescribing, I had never once cured a patient. Now people are cured every week in my practice. As I mentioned, my patients are my partners. We collaborate, and they work hard. They work hard at a time when they feel they can't even lift a finger—when the prospect of walking to the drugstore with a slip of paper twinkles like the North Star in their dark sky. They follow my lead because they feel inspired by my conviction and hope in this new model—one that asks the question "Why?" and has the goal of not only symptom relief but an incredible boost in their vitality.

I realize that many of you reading this book may fear the change that will happen if you take my advice seriously. But no situation has ever been more easily resolved, better handled, or supported by freaking out. Responding with fear leads us to make decisions that are myopic. Some of these decisions may ease our sense of disorder, but they simultaneously engender new and more complex problems. Instead, when you have a symptom—when you feel cloudy, sad, sore, gassy, weepy, tired, or unnecessarily anxious—bring some wonder to it. Ask why and try to make the connections. Your body's symptoms are telling you something about equilibrium. Your body is trying to tell you that it has lost balance. Stand back and appreciate the infinite complexity of your organism. Know that fear will only drive you to treat your body like a robotic machine that needs oil and gear changes. We are so much more than buttons and levers.

So it's time to put on some new glasses and start to study your body. Start to think critically about what you buy, the medical advice you take, and what the media tells you to worry about. Let light shine on every dark corner of your beliefs about health. This critical thinking will liberate you to realize your full potential as a parent, spouse, or friend, and within your own sphere of existence. As one of my favorite quotes goes: "Everything you've ever wanted is on the other side of fear."

In the rest of this chapter, we're going to take a tour of what depression is—from its true definition and biology to its myriad causes and the colossal failure of the pharmaceutical industry to treat this health challenge that has swiftly become the leading cause of disability in America and the rest of the world.[11] This will help ease your fears about the change that you're about to make and set the stage for the balance of the book. And I'll start with one of the most pervasive and harmful myths about depression.

DEPRESSION IS NOT A DISEASE[12]

Psychiatry, unlike other fields of medicine, is based on a highly subjective diagnostic system. Essentially you sit in the office with a physician and you are labeled based on the doctor's opinion of the symptoms you describe. There are no tests. You can't pee in a cup or give a drop of blood to be analyzed for a substance that definitely indicates "you have depression" much in the way a blood test can tell you that you have diabetes or are anemic.

Psychiatry is infamous for saying "oops!" It has a long history of abusing patients with pseudoscience-driven treatments and has been sullied by its shameful lack of diagnostic rigor. Consider, for example, the 1949 Nobel Prize winner Egas Moniz, a Portuguese neurologist who introduced invasive surgical techniques to treat people with schizophrenia by cutting connections between their prefrontal region and other parts of the brain (i.e., the prefrontal lobotomy). And then we had the Rosenhan experiment in the 1970s, which exposed how difficult it is for a doctor to distinguish between an "insane patient" and a sane patient acting insane. Today's prescription pads for psychotropic drugs are, in my belief, just as harmful and absurd as physically destroying critical brain tissue or labeling people as "psychiatric" when really they are anything but.

My fellowship training was in consultation-liaison psychiatry, or "psychosomatic medicine." I was drawn to this specialization because it seemed to be the only one that acknowledged physical processes and pathologies that could manifest behaviorally. I noticed that psychiatrists in this field appreciated the role of biological actions such as inflammation and the stress response. When I watched fellow psychiatrists consult on surgical patients in the hospital, they talked about these processes much differently from when they saw patients in their Park Avenue offices. They talked about delirium brought on by electrolyte imbalance, symptoms of dementia caused by B_{12} deficiency, and the onset of psychosis in someone who was recently prescribed antinausea medication. These root causes of mental challenges are far from the "it's all in your head" banter that typically swirls around conversations about mental illness.

The word *psychosomatic* is a loaded and stigmatized term that implies "it's all in your head." Psychiatry remains the wastebasket for the shortcomings of conventional medicine in terms of diagnosing and treating. If doctors can't explain your symptoms, or if the treatment doesn't fix the problem and further testing doesn't identify a concrete diagnosis, you'll probably be referred to a psychiatrist or, more likely, be handed a prescription for an antidepressant by your family doctor. If you are *very persistent* that you still need real help, your doctor might throw an antipsychotic at you as well. Most prescriptions for antidepressants are doled out by family doctors—not psychiatrists, with 7 percent of all visits to a primary-care doctor ending with an antidepressant prescription.[13] And almost three-quarters of the prescriptions are written without a specific diagnosis.[14] What's more, when the Department of Mental Health at Johns Hopkins Bloomberg School of Public Health did its own examination into the prevalence of mental disorders, it found that "Many individuals who are prescribed and use antidepressant medications may not have met criteria for mental disorders. Our data indicate that antidepressants are commonly used in the absence of clear evidence-based indications."[15]

I'll never forget a case I consulted on several years ago that involved "psychosomatic" facial burning in a woman. Her story is insightful. She complained of an intense burning sensation in her face, though there was no explanation for it other than it being "all in her head." Her symptoms were so disabling that she was barely able to function. I was still prescribing psychotropics at the time, but a voice inside of me knew there was something real going on, and it wasn't at all in her head. But unfortunately the Western medical model had already labeled her as being a psychosomatic case, which called for psychiatric medication and couldn't appreciate or even begin to understand the complexity of her condition. Antidepressants and benzodiazepines (tranquilizers including Valium or Xanax) didn't help her. What ultimately did was dietary change, supplementation, and rebalancing of her bodily flora. Was this all a placebo effect? Clearly she wanted to feel better with such intensity that she would have done anything. But traditional medication didn't cure her. At the heart of her pain and distress was an immune and inflammatory process that could not be remedied via antidepressants and antianxiety drugs. It was fixed through strategies that got to the core of her problem—that yanked the nail out of her foot and let the injury heal.

The idea that depression and all of its relatives are manifestations of glitches in the immune system and inflammatory pathways—not a neurochemical deficiency disorder—is a topic we will explore at length throughout this book. This fact is not as new as you might think, but it's probably not something your general doctor or even psychiatrist will talk about when you complain of symptoms and are hurried out of the office with a prescription for an antidepressant. Nearly a century ago, scientific researchers were already exploring a connection between toxic conditions in the gut and mood and brain function. This phenomenon was given the name *auto intoxication*. But studying such a wild idea fell out of fashion. By mid-century no one was looking into how intestinal health could affect mental health. Instead, the thinking was quickly becoming the reverse—that depression and anxiety influenced the gut. And as the pharmaceutical industry took off in the second half of the twentieth century, gut theories were ignored and the brilliant researchers behind them were forgotten. The gut was regarded as the seat of health in ancient medical practices for centuries; now we can finally appreciate the validity of such old wisdom. Hippocrates, the father of medicine, who lived in the third century BCE, was among the first to say that "all disease begins in the gut."

A multitude of studies now shows an undeniable link between gut dysfunction and the brain, chiefly by revealing the relationship between the volume of inflammatory markers in the blood (i.e., signs of inflammation) and risk for depression.[16] Higher levels of inflammatory markers, which often indicate that the body's immune system is on high alert, significantly increase the risk of developing depression. And these levels parallel the depth of the depression: higher levels equates with more severe depression. Which ultimately means that depression should be categorized with other inflammatory disorders including heart disease, arthritis, multiple sclerosis, diabetes, cancer, and dementia. And it's no surprise, at least to me, that depression is far more common in people with other inflammatory and autoimmune issues like irritable bowel syndrome, chronic fatigue syndrome, fibromyalgia, insulin resistance, and obesity. All of these conditions are characterized by higher levels of inflammation, a topic we'll get into in Chapter 3.

To really grasp the fact that depression is not a disorder primarily rooted in the brain, look no further than some of the most demonstrative studies. When scientists purposefully trigger inflammation in the bodies of healthy people who exhibit no signs of depression by injecting them with a substance (more on this shortly), they quickly develop classic symptoms of depression.[17] And when people with hepatitis C are treated with the pro-inflammatory drug interferon, as many as 45 percent of those individuals develop major depression.[18]

So when people ask me about why we're suffering from what appears to be an epidemic of depression despite the number of people taking antidepressants, I don't think about brain chemistry. I turn to the impact of our sedentary lifestyles, processed food diets, and unrelenting stress. I turn to the medical literature that says a typical Western diet—high in refined carbs, unnatural fats, and foods that create chaos in our blood sugar balance—contribute to higher levels of inflammation.[19] Contrary to what you might assume, one of the most influential risk factors for depression is high blood sugar. Most people view diabetes and depression as two distinct conditions, but new scientific findings are rewriting the textbooks. One game-changing study published in 2010 that followed more than 65,000 women over a decade showed that women with diabetes were nearly 30 percent more likely to develop depression.[20] This heightened risk remained even after the researchers excluded other risk factors such as lack of physical exercise and weight. Moreover, diabetic women who took insulin were 53 percent more likely to develop depression.

Certainly you can draw the same conclusions that I've made: the rates of diabetes have skyrocketed alongside those of depression in the past two decades. And so have the rates of obesity, which is also correlated with increased inflammatory markers. Studies show that obesity is associated with a 55 percent increased risk of depression, and it cuts the other way too: depression is associated with a 58 percent increased risk of developing obesity.[21] In the cogent words of a group of Australian researchers in a 2013 paper: "A range of factors appear to increase the risk for the development of depression and seem to be associated with systemic inflammation; these include psychosocial stressors, poor diet, physical inactivity, obesity, smoking, altered gut [function], [allergies], dental [cavities], sleep and vitamin D deficiency."[22]

In 2014 Scottish researchers addressed the gap between what the science says about the causes of depression and what patients experience when they find themselves caught in the default web of psychiatric care. In their paper they highlight the value of what I practice: psychoneuroimmunology.[23] Indeed, it's a mouthful of a word, but it simply refers to examining (and respecting) the complex interplay between various systems and organs of the body, especially those that syncopate the nervous, gastrointestinal, and immune systems in a brilliant dance that in turn affects mental well-being. These researchers point out that many patients who are told they have psychiatric conditions originating in their head or related to some (fictitious) brain chemical deficiency actually share real biological imbalances related to their immune-inflammatory pathways. These patients show elevated levels of inflammatory markers in their blood, signs that their body is on the defensive, activating processes that can result in unexplainable physical symptoms and that are diagnosed as psychiatric rather than biologic. And rather than treating the underlying biology, they are instead relegated to a lifetime of therapy and medication, to no avail.

The conditions examined by these researchers were depression, chronic fatigue, and "somatization," the latter of which is what we call the production of symptoms with no plausible organic cause. These diagnoses have a lot in common in terms of symptoms: fatigue, sensitivity to pain, inability to concentrate, flu-like malaise, and cognitive issues. Isn't it interesting that each of these conditions is often diagnosed as a separate illness and yet they share so much in common from a biological standpoint? As the authors state: "If psychiatry is to rise to the challenge of being a science, then it must respond to the [existing] data in reconceptualizing boundaries. As such, the data reviewed here challenge the organizational power structures in psychiatry."[24]

Personalized lifestyle medicine that accounts for the role of the environment in triggering inflammation and the manipulation of the immune and endocrine systems is the most sensible way to approach those individuals who would otherwise be candidates for multiple medications. It turns out that it may not all be in your head—but rather in the interconnectedness among the gut, immune, and endocrine systems.

In upcoming chapters, we're going to be exploring all of these connections—the indelible links between your gut and its microbial inhabitants, your immune system, and the orchestra of hormones that course through your body in sync with a day-night cycle. These connections influence the state of your entire physiology and, as important, your mental health and overall sense of well-being. While it may seem odd to talk about the gut-based immune system in terms of mental health, the latest science reveals that it may be the body's—and mind's—center of gravity. Just as

I write this, yet another new study has emerged that overturns decades of textbook teaching about the brain and immune system. Researchers at the University of Virginia School of Medicine have determined that the brain is directly connected to the immune system by lymphatic vessels we didn't know existed.[25] That we had no idea about these vessels given the fact that the lymphatic system has been so thoroughly studied and charted throughout the body is astonishing on its own. And such a discovery will have significant effects on the study and treatment of neurological diseases, from autism and multiple sclerosis to Alzheimer's disease and, yes, depression. It's time we rewrite the textbooks. And it's time we treat depression for what it really is.

So if depression isn't a disease, then what is it? As I briefly mentioned in the introduction, depression is a *symptom,* a vague surface sign at best that doesn't tell you anything about its root cause. Consider, for a moment, that your toe hurts. Any number of things can cause a toe to hurt, from physically injuring it to a bunion, blister, or tumor growing inside. The hurting is a sign that something is wrong with the toe, simple as that. Likewise, depression is the hurting; it's an adaptive response, intelligently communicated by the body, to something not being right within, often because things are also off in our environment.

Depression doesn't always manifest with feelings of serious melancholy and sadness or the urge to sit on the couch all day brooding. I can't even remember the last patient I saw who was like the person you see on a TV commercial for an antidepressant. All of my patients experience anxiety—an inner kinetic discomfort, restlessness, unease, and a lot of insomnia. In fact, most cases of depression involve women who are very much on the go and productive, but they are also anxious, scatterbrained, overly stressed out, irritable, forgetful, worrywarts, unable to concentrate, and feeling "wired and tired" at the same time. And many of them have been dismissed by the medical system; their psychiatric problems were created by mistreatment as they fell into the vortex of endless prescription medications.

Take, for another example, a forty-two-year-old patient of mine we'll call Jane, who fell into this black hole after being treated for irritable bowel and acne with drugs, including the now discontinued Accutane (isotretinoin). Jane experienced a depressed mood, a common side effect of Accutane, and was then put on an antidepressant as she stopped the medication (isotretinoin is a retinoid, a strong medication used to treat severe acne; it causes birth defects in babies born from mothers who take it during pregnancy, so it's carefully regulated and only available in its generic form under a special program). After the death of her parents, which triggered more symptoms of depression, Jane was diagnosed with a thyroid problem, and her doctor at the time prescribed radioablation therapy, which destroys thyroid tissue with radioactive iodine 131. This led to her having acute panic attacks, and she soon began taking Xanax. Symptoms of more thyroid problems, including brain fog, extreme fatigue, and physical pain, culminated in a diagnosis of fibromyalgia. Jane was then treated with birth control pills and an antibiotic and soon developed chronic yeast infections, bloating, and abdominal pain. By the time she came to me, Jane had a twenty-four-hour home health aide.

Jane's experience reflects that of so many people labeled as depressed and sent away with yet another prescription. The system creates patients who are otherwise healthy and just need to recalibrate their bodies using simple lifestyle interventions, mostly around diet—not drugs. After all, it is through diet that we communicate with our environment. It's a dialect that we've forgotten how to speak.

AN EVOLUTIONARY MISMATCH

Take a look around you and appreciate the world we live in today with its technologies and conveniences: computers, cars, cell phones, and supermarkets. But also consider the mismatch between this scenario and the days when we had to forage for our food and sleep under the stars. Our caveman days are still very much a part of our DNA because evolution is slow; what seems like ages in cultural time (20,000 years ago) is but a blink of an eye in biological time. Which brings me to ask the question: Is all this depression simply a sign of an *evolutionary mismatch*?

This is the term that encompasses the source of most modern ills. We are engaged in lifestyles that are not compatible with what our genome has evolved over millions of years to expect. We eat a poor diet, harbor too much stress, lack sufficient physical movement, deprive ourselves of natural sunlight, expose ourselves to environmental toxicants, and take too many pharmaceuticals. Our wayward departure is marked by two specific revolutions in the history of mankind: the Neolithic, or agricultural, Revolution and the Industrial Revolution. For 99 percent of our existence, we followed the so-called Paleolithic diet, which is devoid of inflammatory and "insulinotropic" foods like sugar, grains, and dairy. Our body's microbial ecology has been one of the primary victims of this shift—the 90 percent of our cells that are non-human in nature and that account for the majority of our body's activities, which in turn impact the expression of our genes. I'll be going into greater depth about the human microbiome in Chapter 3, but I'll give you a short primer here because this discussion is important and will be carried throughout the book.

Although we've learned to think of bacteria as agents of death for the most part because certain strains can cause lethal infections in compromised hosts, new science is compelling us to consider how some of these microscopic bugs are fundamental to life—and mental health. As you read this, some 100 trillion microbes are colonized in your intestines alone.[26] They outnumber your own cells by a factor of about ten, covering your insides and outsides. And they contain estimates of more than 8 million genes of their own, which means that *fully 99 percent of the genetic material in your body is not your own. It belongs to your microbial comrades.* These microbes not only influence the expression of our DNA, but research reveals that throughout our evolution microbial DNA has become part of our own DNA. In other words, genes from microbes have inserted themselves into our genetic code (mitochondrial DNA being the prime example) to help us evolve and flourish.

A great many of these invisible creatures live within your digestive tract, and while they include fungi, parasites, and viruses, it's the bacteria that appear to hold the proverbial keys to the kingdom of your biology, as they support every conceivable feature of your health. In the future we'll likely see how the other microbes contribute at least as much to our health as bacteria do. The microbiome is so crucial to human health that it could be considered an organ in and of itself. In fact, it has been suggested that since without it we could not live, we should consider ourselves a "meta-organism," inseparable from it. This inner ecology helps you digest food and absorb nutrients, supports the immune system and the body's detoxification pathways, produces and releases important enzymes and substances that collaborate with your biology (including chemicals for the brain, such as vitamins and neurotransmitters), helps you handle stress through its effects on your endocrine—hormonal—system, and even ensures you get a good night's sleep. Put simply, your microbiome influences practically everything about your health, including how you feel both emotionally, physically, and mentally.

What compromises a healthy microbiome? Not surprisingly, your microbiome is vulnerable to three antagonizing forces: exposure to substances that kill or otherwise negatively change the composition of the bacterial colonies (these substances include everything from environmental chemicals and drugs like antibiotics to ingredients such as artificial sugars and processed gluten-containing foods); a lack of nutrients that support healthy, diverse tribes of good microbes; and unrelenting stress.

I've devoted an entire section to the amazing features of the microbiome, so you'll gain plenty of knowledge about how it plays a role in your physical and mental well-being and how you can maintain an optimal colony of tribes. We have coevolved with these microorganisms throughout our journey on this planet, and we must respect them for what they are: the body's—and brain's—best friend. And they are as much a part of our survival and mental well-being as our own cells are.

DESIGNED FOR DEPRESSION

Have you ever stopped to wonder if depression has benefits? I know, it sounds a little outlandish to even suggest such an idea. But it's an excellent question to ask and an even better one to answer. This conversation, however, is best couched within the topic of stress in general. So let's go there next.

Most of us can recognize the symptoms of stress. We feel it inside and out. We become irritable, our heart races, our face may feel hot, we get a familiar headache or upset stomach, our mind is incessantly chattering, there's a sense of impending doom, and we're annoyed by the smallest things. For some people, stress has little outward effect. For these individuals, what they feel at the surface is internalized and sometimes expressed as disease. In fact, many of these people don't believe they experience stress—but they do; they just don't consciously recognize it until it builds up to a certain point and seeps out in other ways.

The term *stress* as it is used today was coined by one of the founding fathers of stress research, Hans Selye, who in 1936 defined it as "the non-specific response of the body to any demand for change."[27] Selye proposed that when subjected to persistent stress, both humans and animals could develop certain life-threatening afflictions such as heart attack or stroke that previously were thought to be caused by specific pathogens only. This is a crucial point, because it demonstrates the impact that everyday life and experiences have not only on our emotional well-being but also on our physical health.

The word *stress* as it relates to emotions became part of our vocabulary in the 1950s. Its use became common with the onset of the Cold War, which was an era when fear ruled. We were frightened of atomic war, so we built bomb shelters. As a society, we could not say we were afraid; instead, we used the word *stress*. Today we continue to use the word to describe anything that disrupts us emotionally—we're stressed, stressed out, under stress, and so on. Stress can also be described as the thoughts, feelings, behaviors, and physiological changes that happen when we respond to demands and perceptions. And if those demands placed on us overwhelm our perceived ability to cope, we experience "stress." In our frenzied minds, we begin to pant silently like an animal and look for an escape.

Since Selye, researchers have broken stress down into several subcategories. Stress physiology has come a long way in the last fifty years in particular, and so have the stressors. A key concept to enter the medical vernacular more recently is what is known as allostatic load. Your allostatic load refers to environmental challenges—the "wear and tear" on the body—that cause it to begin efforts to maintain stability (allostasis, also known as homeostasis). It also represents the physiological consequences of adapting to chronic stress that entails repeated activation of the body's stress response machinery involving many systems—immune, endocrine, and neuronal. Researchers Bruce McEwen and Eliot Stellar coined this term in 1993 as a more precise alternative to the term *stress*.[28] The key players of the stress response, cortisol and epinephrine (adrenaline), have both protective and adverse effects on the body depending on when and how much they are used. On one hand, these hormones are essential for the body's ability to adapt and maintain balance (homeostasis), but if they are flowing for a prolonged period or needed relatively frequently, they can accelerate disease processes. The allostatic load, as it's called, becomes more harmful than helpful. This load can be measured in physiological systems as chemical imbalances in the activities of the nervous, hormonal, and immune systems. It can also be measured by disturbances in the body's day-night cycle (what's called the circadian rhythm, another concept we'll explore later), and in some cases, changes to the brain's physical structure.

Stress is actually a good thing, at least from an evolutionary and survivalist perspective. It serves an important function: to protect us from real danger by equipping us with a better means to escape a life-threatening situation or face it head on. But our physical reaction doesn't change according to the type or magnitude of a perceived threat. Whether it's a truly perilous stressor, or just the to-do list and an argument with a colleague, the body's stress response is the same. Let me give you a quick lesson on what goes on when your body senses stress so we can come full circle back to, dare I say, the secret value of depression.

First, the brain sends a message to the adrenal glands that results in the release of adrenaline, also called epinephrine. This triggers your heart rate to increase as blood is directed to your muscles in the event you need to flee. When the threat is gone, your body normalizes again. But if the threat doesn't go away and your stress response intensifies, then a series of events take place along what's called the HPA axis, short for hypothalamic-pituitary-adrenal axis, and which involves multiple stress hormones. The hypothalamus is a small but key governing region of the brain that has a vital role in controlling many bodily functions, including the release of hormones from the pituitary gland housed inside. It's often referred to as the seat of our emotions because it commands much of our emotional processing. The moment you feel nervous, anxious, extremely overwhelmed, or simply worried that you can't deal with life, the hypothalamus releases a corticotropin-releasing hormone (CRH), a substance that starts a cascade of reactions, ending with cortisol flowing into your bloodstream. While this process has been well defined for a long time, newer research reveals that perceptions of stress trigger inflammatory signaling from the body to travel to the brain, priming it for hyper-response.[29]

You're probably already familiar with cortisol, the body's main stress hormone that aids in that famous fight-or-flight response. It also controls how your body processes carbohydrates, fats, and proteins. Because it's the hormone responsible for protecting you during times of stress, its actions increase your appetite, promote more fat storage, and break down complex molecules and tissues that can be used for quick forms of energy, including muscle. For this reason, continual exposure to excess cortisol over time can lead to increased abdominal fat, bone loss, a suppressed immune system, fatigue, and a heightened risk for insulin resistance, diabetes, heart disease, and full-blown depression. Cortisol does, however, serve a positive role. It directs and buffers the immune system and primes the body for attack. This would all be great if the attack were short-lived and easily resolved. The attack of our modern-day lifestyles is unrelenting.

The scientific study of the impact of stress on the body from the inside out, and even the outside in, has made tremendous advances in the fifteen years starting in 1998 when Harvard University researchers conducted a joint study with several Boston-area hospitals designed to examine the interactions between the mind and the body, specifically the skin. They called their discovery the NICE (neuro-immuno-cutaneous-endocrine) network.[30] In plain speak, it's a giant interactive network consisting of your nervous system, immune system, the skin, and your endocrine (hormonal) system. All of these are intimately connected through a dialogue of a complex array of biochemicals.

The Boston researchers studied how various external forces influence our state of mind, from massage and aromatherapy to depression and isolation. What they discovered confirmed what many in the scientific community have known anecdotally for centuries: our state of mind has a definite impact on our health and even our appearance. People suffering from depression, for example, often look older than their chronological age. They don't appear healthy and vibrant, as the stress of coping with depression has accelerated the aging process and damaged their health.

Since the NICE network entered our vocabulary, dozens of other studies have been performed to confirm the powerful interplay between psychology and biology or, put simply, mind over matter. An analogy I like to use in my practice goes like this: If you're walking down a dark alleyway at night and hear footsteps behind you, you might be alerted in uncomfortable ways, and your body will prepare to fight or flee. But if you then hear your friend's voice, everything in your body's physiology changes in that one instant. Yet the only thing that's changed is your perception!

So going back to the question "Can depression be good for us?" Was depression once an adaptive response to the environment? I subscribe to the idea that the body doesn't make mistakes after millions of years of evolution. A 2014 review in the *Journal of Affective Disorders* attempts to answer the question of why we get depressed, rather than just looking at how, and what to do about it. Often the best approach to root cause resolution of symptoms comes from an understanding of the reasons why the body is responding in the way that it is. Speaking to the concept of evolutionary mismatch, the authors of the paper state: ". . . modern humans exist in environments that are critically different from those in which we evolved, and that our new environments interact with our ancient genomes to lead to disorder . . ."[31]

The authors discuss how depression may have served a purpose at some point, but the nature and intensity of today's modern-day triggers may be leaving more of us depressed (up to 41 percent of us!) more of the time than seems reasonable. This perspective encompasses the inflammatory model of depression, which posits that both psychological stress and bodily inflammation result in brain-based changes that would serve us if they were brief, but may kill us if they are persistent (something like that).

The researchers of the review go on to explain how antidepressants are missing the mark, and why their prescription should be reconsidered, citing side effects including:

> . . . headache, nausea, insomnia, sexual dysfunction, agitation, sedation, hyponatremia, stroke, cardiac conduction defects, and increased risk of mortality. The long-term use of antidepressants may be associated with additional adverse effects. For instance, some antidepressants may be weakly carcinogenic or cause osteoporosis. Antidepressants have also been associated with an increased acute risk of suicide in younger patients while they may decrease the risk of suicide

in older patients or with longer-term use. Also, all major classes of antidepressants have been associated with unpleasant (and sometimes dangerous) symptoms when they are discontinued abruptly. Discontinuation of antidepressants is associated with relapse and recurrence of MDD (Major Depressive Disorder). In a meta-analysis, this risk was shown to be higher for antidepressants that cause greater disruption to neurotransmitter systems . . . [And] there is a growing body of research suggesting that when they are used in the long term as a maintenance treatment, antidepressants can lose efficacy, and may even result in chronic and treatment-resistant depression. Such reactions may be due to the brain's attempt to maintain homeostasis and a functioning adaptation in spite of the medication.

For someone like me, this is a profound summary of the perspectives I have curated since my departure from conventional practice. The call to action is to view depression as the vague descriptive term that it is. Put simply, depression is a sign for us to stop and figure out what's causing our imbalance. Another way to appreciate this perspective is to say *depression is an opportunity.*

Many of my patients are initially surprised to experience my wrath about the prescribing that's going on all around me. I don't think New York is any different from Anytown USA in how heavy-handed the average practitioner, whether it's a family practice doctor or an internist or psychiatrist, is with prescriptions. In my opinion, it has become reckless. Their patients have never consented to the long-term effects of these medications because pharmaceutical research is, by nature, short term.[32] There's no incentive on the part of the pharmaceutical companies to take a good look at what happens to the average individual when she takes a medication for a decade or so. That said, in recent years there's been a spat of studies linking antidepressants to an increased risk of aggression, homicide, and suicide, as well as fingers pointed at these drugs for their involvement in school shootings, airplane crashes, and other unfortunate events often blamed on terrorists, gun access, or *lack* of treatment.[33]

In one particularly alarming paper published in 2015 in no less an authority than the *British Medical Journal,* researchers from the Nordic Cochrane Centre, an independent drug safety analysis group based in Denmark, found that more than half a million people aged sixty-five and older in the West die every year from psych meds.[34] Using an impressive meta-analysis of placebo-controlled trials, these researchers discovered that more patients die from taking FDA-approved antidepressants than do patients who take no drugs or who use other unconventional treatment methods. Similarly, the all-cause mortality rate (translation: dying from any cause) was found to be 3.6 percent higher among patients who take newly approved antidepressants compared to patients who take no antidepressants. The study's scientists highlighted the fact most industry-funded studies favoring psych meds tend to skew the sample groups and test data so much that the results end up becoming meaningless. Underreporting of deaths, according to the study's authors, is another major problem in the clinical trial process. The Nordic group estimates that the suicide rate among antidepressant users is some fifteen times higher than what the Food and Drug Administration (FDA) reports publicly.

Studies like this that uncover our modern medical assault on humanity are just the tip of the proverbial iceberg. I could write a whole book on the high-profile research demonstrating that patients are held hostage by psychiatric medications, made sicker, and convinced that neither is true. They are more likely to experience a worsening of their depression, as these drugs have been proven in rigorous studies to be mood destabilizers (contrary to what conventional wisdom says).[35] I should also add that they've recently been labeled as carcinogens.[36] In a major review published by the *Australian and New Zealand Journal of Psychiatry,* a group of researchers from a variety of institutions including Tufts University, Harvard University, and the University of Parma in Italy reported that the vast majority of psychotropic drugs can cause cancer in animals.[37]

Although the animal-based results are not enough to draw definitive conclusions in humans, these same animal studies are often used to justify drug and chemical safety, and therefore they are enough to warrant caution and appropriate informed consent. Unfortunately, these conversations are not happening.

Don't panic if you're taking an antidepressant now.

The information in this book will help you take control of this symptom once and for all, and if tapering is right for you, I'll be sharing my personal guide for doing just that in Chapter 10. For now, accept the fact that we are all designed for depression as humans. It can be a warning sign that something isn't right within. And just as we are designed to feel glum, we are also designed to self-heal and feel great.

DEPRESSION ISN'T GENETIC, IT'S EPIGENETIC

One of my favorite practice-changing papers was a 2003 case report of a lifelong vegetarian who experienced a month and a half of progressively worsening depression.[38] Eventually she began to hear voices and feel paranoid. The fifty-two-year-old postmenopausal woman ultimately became what's called catatonic, which meant she was awake and alive but nonresponsive, and largely in an otherwise vegetative state. One would automatically assume this was a serious case of severe pathology. She was treated with electroconvulsive therapy and antipsychotics to no avail. And then she was transferred to another hospital, where they happened to test her levels of vitamin B_{12}. They found that she was a tad on the low side, and after receiving a vitamin B_{12} injection, she fully recovered. Coincidence? I think not. While it may be one of the more extreme cases, it's emblematic of how a simple but critical deficiency can be at the causal root of psychiatric manifestations. Later on, we'll see how vitamin B_{12} deficiency has long been implicated in the development of depression. It's a classic example of how we are not just puppets at the mercy of our encoded DNA, but rather products of the complex interactions between our genes and our environment. And it's now well established that our health outcomes are dominated more by our environment than our inheritance. As I like to remind my patients, depression is *epigenetic*, not genetic.

Even though genes encoded by DNA are more or less static (barring the occurrence of mutation), the expression of those genes can be highly dynamic in response to environmental influences. This field of study, called epigenetics, is now one of the hottest areas of research. Epigenetics, defined more technically, is the study of sections of your DNA (called "marks," or "markers") that essentially tell your genes when and how strongly to express themselves. Like conductors of an orchestra, these epigenetic marks control not only your health and longevity, but also how you pass your genes on to future generations. Indeed, the forces acting on the expression of your DNA today can be passed on to your future biological children, affecting how their genes behave in their lives and whether or not *their* children will face a higher risk of certain diseases and disorders, depression included. But, by the same token, these marks can be changed to read differently, making it fully possible to *reverse* certain diseases.

We in the scientific community believe epigenetic forces affect us from our days in utero until the day we die. There are likely many windows during our lifetime when we are sensitive to environmental impacts that can change our biology and have major downstream effects such as symptoms of depression. At the same time, the multitude of neural, immune, and hormonal actions that are controlled by the microbiome—and that in turn command our entire physiology—are susceptible to disruption and adaptation, especially by environmental changes.

One of the most important takeaways from this first chapter is to understand that depression is not about the brain per se. Of course, there are brain events and biochemical reactions occurring when a person feels depressed, but no research has ever established that a particular brain state causes, or even correlates with, depression. Many different physical conditions create psychiatric symptoms but aren't themselves psychiatric. We think (because our doctors think) that we need to "cure" the brain, but in reality we need to look at the whole body's ecosystem: intestinal health, hormonal interactions, the immune system and autoimmune disorders, blood sugar balance, and toxicant exposure. And we need natural, evidence-based alternatives to psychiatric medications—treatments that target what's really awry in our bodies. That means strategic dietary supplementation and noninvasive remedies like light therapy and cranial stimulation, but also smart (i.e., biologically compatible) food protocols and exercise choices, restful sleep, a detoxed environment, and meditation/relaxation practices. The best way to heal our brains is to heal the bodies in which they reside. Or, as I also like to put it, free your mind by healing your whole body. Hence the whole purpose of this book. The potential for lifestyle-based interventions and healing is immense.

When I get asked about the main triggers of depression, I often think of the three types of patients I generally see: the woman with blood sugar issues and nutritional deficiencies due to the standard American diet (high in sugar, low in healthy fats); the individual with a misbehaving thyroid, which plays into all matters of hormones that in turn affect mental health; and the person with either medication-induced depression (think statins, birth control pills, proton-pump inhibitors like Nexium and Prilosec, and even vaccines). We're going to be exploring all of these potential triggers in detail in the upcoming chapters.

Although scientists are now trying to identify drivers of different types of depressive syndromes, the medical industry still offers a one-size-fits-all solution (read: one drug, one disorder model). This is akin to studying all the different sources of, say, back pain—from a torn muscle or a herniated disc to cancer or a kidney infection—but using the same treatment protocol on all cases. It doesn't make sense, and there can be unintended consequences if that singular treatment entails risky drugs or surgery. And when it comes to using antidepressants for all signs of depression, this can be very tricky terrain, as the next chapter shows.

CHAPTER 2

Truth Serum: Coming Clean About the Serotonin Myth

How You've Been Misled, Misdiagnosed, and Mistreated

There's no such thing as an antidepressant.

⸺

The chemical imbalance theory of depression is heavily promoted but remains unfounded.

D o you take antidepressants? Do you know someone who does? Maybe you even have friends and family members who swear they have been lifesaving. Antidepressants might seem like a reasonable option, particularly if things are dire. But do you know the whole story?

At the risk of sounding extreme, let me give you an example from my own case files that sets the tone for this chapter. Kate had never been on an antidepressant and never suffered from depression, but she felt overwhelmed and frazzled after the birth of her first baby. At her six-week postpartum follow-up appointment, her obstetrician prescribed Zoloft. Within one week of starting it, she had written a suicide note and was planning to jump off of her fifteenth-floor Manhattan balcony. She said to me, "It just made sense at the time. And I felt really detached about it, like it was nothing."

Kate's experience is not an outlier. She is among millions of women who are reflexively prescribed medication for symptoms of distress. She's also among those who have serious side effects that may seem like part of the depression—not a result of the drugs. Rather than examining the sources of her postpartum plight, Kate found herself in dangerously unfamiliar territory in the name of treatment. If only she had known the whole story before deciding to fill that prescription.

The ease with which these medications are dispensed is partly why so many take them: 11 percent of all Americans, 25 percent of whom are women in their forties and fifties. The use of anti-depressants has increased almost 400 percent from 1998 to 2008, making them the third most commonly prescribed drugs across all ages. The sharp increase does not necessarily signify a depression epidemic. Through the early 2000s pharmaceutical companies aggressively tested antidepressants for a variety of disorders, which led to an explosion of FDA-approved uses, from depression to premature ejaculation.[1] Believe it or not, we are spending more on anti-depressants than the gross national product of more than half of the world's countries. Sixty percent of people on antidepressants stay on them for more than two years, and 14 percent do so for more than a decade. By a conservative estimate, 15 percent of *pregnant* women take psychiatric medication today, a rate that has tripled in just the last couple of years.

The medical industry isn't selling a cure. They are selling sickness.

SELLING SICKNESS[2]

Is there a connection between the profligate use of antidepressants and increasing rates of disability? Before antidepressants became so widely used, the National Institute of Mental Health (NIMH) assured people that recovering from a depressive episode was common and that experiencing a second episode was uncommon.[3] But then how do we explain soaring rates of disability and escalating prescriptions?

Robert Whitaker, a notable critic of modern psychiatry and author of *Anatomy of an Epidemic* and *Mad in America,* has compiled and analyzed data showing that days of work lost are not decreased by medication treatment.[4] Much to the contrary, they are *increased* by drug treatment, and so is long-term disability. He also has reported on studies showing that people treated for the illness are three times more likely than the untreated individuals to suffer a "cessation" of their "principal social role," meaning that they function less optimally. And they were nearly seven times more likely to become "incapacitated." Moreover, 85 percent of unmedicated patients recover in a year, with 67 percent doing so by six months.[5] From my perspective, that's an enviable statistic.

What's going on here? In the past half century, the *Diagnostic and Statistical Manual*—the DSM, the bible of diagnosable disorders in psychiatry—has lengthened to more than three hundred diagnoses in its fifth edition. In 1952 the DSM was a slim 130 pages and outlined 106 illnesses. Today's version is a colossal 886 pages and includes 374 diagnoses. It encompasses a general consensus by a committee consisting of practitioners with profound conflicts of interest and pharmaceutical enmeshments.[6] As Dr. Allen Frances of Columbia University and author of *Saving Normal* states: "Wholesale imperial medicalization of normality that will trivialize mental disorder and lead to a deluge of unneeded medication treatment—a bonanza for the pharmaceutical industry but at a huge cost to the new false positive patients caught in the excessively wide DSM-V net."[7] Dr. Frances is the psychiatrist who chaired the task force that produced the fourth edition of the DSM and has been critical of the latest tome. In 2013, Frances rightfully said that "psychiatric diagnosis still relies exclusively on fallible subjective judgments rather than objective biological tests."[8]

When you look at the impossibly long list of symptoms and maladies for which antidepressants can be prescribed, it's practically farcical. These drugs are indicated for classic signs of depression as well as all of the following: premenstrual syndrome, anxiety, obsessive-compulsive disorder (OCD), bipolar disorder, anorexia and binge eating, pain, irritable bowel, and explosive disorders fit for anger management class. Some doctors prescribe them for arthritis, hot flashes, migraine, irritable bowel syndrome, and panic disorder. The fact that antidepressants can be prescribed to treat arthritis, an inflammatory disease of the joints, undermines any beliefs about their ability to precisely correct a chemical imbalance at the root of everything from phobias to bulimia and melancholic depression. The condemning 2015 paper by researchers at Johns Hopkins Bloomberg School of Public Health that I discussed in the previous chapter clearly states that antidepressants are used willy-nilly.[9] In their study, the authors conclude that most people who take antidepressants never meet the medical criteria for a bona fide diagnosis of major depression, and many who are given antidepressants for conditions like OCD, panic disorder, social phobia, and anxiety don't actually have these conditions.

Let's not forget the use of these medications in young children. And they are prescribed not only for depression but behavioral issues such as inattention, temper tantrums, tics, autism, and impaired thinking. How did we ever come to think that this could be a safe and effective treatment for two-year-olds still in diapers who don't even speak in full sentences yet? For starters, consider Study 329, which cost GlaxoSmithKlein $3 billion for their efforts to promote antidepressants to youngsters.[10] This drug company manipulated data that hid signs of increased risk of suicide. The company also falsely represented Paxil as outperforming a placebo.[11]

Among the most celebrated and respected thought leaders in my field is Joanna Moncrieff. She is a senior lecturer in psychiatry at University College London and co-chair of the Critical Psychiatry Network, a group of psychiatrists who dispute the generally accepted model of depression and seek alternative approaches to psychiatry. In a seminal 2006 paper, "Do Antidepressants Cure or

Create Abnormal Brain States?", Moncrieff and her coauthor write: "Our analysis indicates that there are no specific antidepressant drugs, that most of the short-term effects of antidepressants are shared by many other drugs, and that long-term drug treatment with antidepressants or any other drugs has not been shown to lead to long-term elevation of mood. We suggest that the term 'antidepressant' should be abandoned."[12]

At this point, you might be wondering: Where did antidepressants come from and how did they get so popular?

A MEME IS BORN[13]

The predominant theory behind modern antidepressants (SSRIs, or selective serotonin reuptake inhibitors) is that they work by increasing the availability of serotonin, a neurotransmitter famously associated with mood, in the gaps between cells of the brain. In fact, if you were to quiz someone on the street about the biology of depression, they would likely parrot "chemical imbalance" in the brain and go so far as to say a "serotonin deficiency." This hypothesis, referred to as the monoamine hypothesis, grew primarily out of two main observations made in the 1950s and '60s.[14] One was seen in patients being treated for tuberculosis who experienced mood-related side effects from the antitubercular drug iproniazid, which can change the levels of serotonin in the brain. Another was the claim that reserpine, a medication introduced for seizures and high blood pressure, depleted these chemicals and caused depression—that is, until there was a fifty-four person study that demonstrated that it *resolved* depression.[15]

From these preliminary and largely inconsistent observations a theory was born, crystallized by the work and writings of the late Dr. Joseph Schildkraut, who threw fairy dust into the field in 1965 with his speculative manifesto "The Catecholamine Hypothesis of Affective Disorders."[16] Dr. Schildkraut was a prominent psychiatrist at Harvard who studied catecholamines, a class of naturally occurring compounds that act as chemical messengers, or neurotransmitters, within the brain. He looked at one neurochemical in particular, norepinephrine, in people before and during treatment with antidepressants and found that depression suppressed its effectiveness as a chemical messenger. Based on his findings, he theorized broadly about the biochemical underpinnings of mental illnesses. In a field struggling to establish legitimacy (beyond the therapeutic lobotomy!), psychiatry was desperate for a rebranding, and the pharmaceutical industry was all too happy to partner in the effort.

This idea that these medications correct an imbalance that has something to do with a brain chemical has been so universally accepted that no one bothers to question it or even research it using modern rigors of science. According to Dr. Joanna Moncrieff, we have been led to believe that these medications have *disease-based* effects—that they're actually fixing, curing, correcting a real disease in human physiology. Six decades of study, however, have revealed conflicting, confusing, and inconclusive data.[17] That's right: there *has never* been a human study that successfully links low serotonin levels and depression. Imaging studies, blood and urine tests, postmortem suicide assessments, and even animal research have never validated the link between neurotransmitter levels and depression.[18] In other words, *the serotonin theory of depression is a total myth* that has been unjustly supported by the manipulation of data. Much to the contrary, high serotonin levels have been linked to a range of problems, including schizophrenia and autism.[19]

Paul Andrews, an assistant professor of psychology, neuroscience, and behavior at McMaster University in Canada, is among the vocal experts challenging the traditional depression model. In a 2015 review, he declares that the science behind antidepressant medications appears to be backward: serotonin is a downer, not an upper.[20] He argues that serotonin is almost like a first responder to stress. When our bodies are under duress, serotonin helps to reallocate resources at a cellular level. This further shows that we really have no idea what's going on when it comes to looking at one simple chemical. Andrews brings up a good point in a recent review: we can't measure serotonin in a living human brain yet, so it's impossible to know exactly how the brain is releasing and using serotonin. What scientists must do instead is rely on evidence about levels of serotonin that the brain has already metabolized, and by studying seratonin in animal models. To date, the best available evidence indicates that *more* serotonin—not less—is released and used during depressive episodes. This natural surge of serotonin helps the brain adapt to depression; it forces the body to spend more energy on conscious thought than to areas such as growth, development, reproduction, immune function, and the stress response.[21]

Andrews also happens to be an evolutionary psychologist, and has asserted in previous research that antidepressants leave individuals worse off after they stop taking them. He agrees that even though depression can be a painful, troubling experience, most forms of depression are normal adaptations to stress. According to Andrews, when patients on SSRI medication improve, it appears that their brains are actually *overcoming the effects of antidepressants, rather than being helped by them.* The drugs are interfering with the brain's own mechanisms of recovery. This is an important point, because time and time again people ask me how antidepressants appear to be helpful in the short term. Perhaps, in the rare instance that their effects are adaptive, it is by virtue of the brain's own powers trying to combat the assault of the antidepressants—not the other way around. But over time, as the assault continues, the brain is functionally compromised under the constant force of the incoming drugs.

One critical review of the serotonin hypothesis concludes: " . . . there is no direct evidence of serotonin or norepinephrine deficiency despite thousands of studies that have attempted to validate this notion."[22] And in a scathing review on major depression published in the *New England Journal of Medicine* in 2008, the researchers write: ". . . numerous studies of norepinephrine and serotonin metabolites in plasma, urine, and cerebrospinal fluid as well as postmortem studies of the brains of patients with depression, have yet to identify the purported deficiency reliably."[23]

In the cogent words of Dr. Daniel Carlat, author of *Unhinged,* "We have convinced ourselves that we have developed cures for mental illnesses . . . when in fact we know so little about the underlying neurobiology of their causes that our treatments are often a series of trials and errors."[24] Indeed, the brain orchestrates a delicate interplay among some one hundred neurotransmitters, including fourteen different types of serotonin receptors. To think we can cherry-pick one brain chemical and cure all and every behavioral disturbance is a gross oversimplification and downright absurd.

The brain is much more complex than the serotonin model can describe. To be clear, SSRIs block the removal of serotonin from the junctions between nerve cells (synapses) in the brain so there's increased firing of serotonin nerves. But when serotonergic nerves are overstimulated, they become less sensitive in a bid to establish equilibrium again. In science speak this is called downregulation. And such downregulation doesn't return to normal after the drug is stopped. We in the scientific community still don't know if the downregulation can become permanent, but a cadre of my colleagues and I believe this poses a serious risk to the brain. It's no surprise to me that in the first twelve years after its initial marketing blitz, Prozac was named in more than 40,000 reports of adverse effects submitted to the FDA.[25] No other drug comes close to such a history.

Even if we accepted the proposition that these drugs are helpful for some people, extrapolating a medical cause from this observation would be akin to saying that shyness is caused by a deficiency of alcohol, or that headaches are caused by a lack of codeine. And what about a genetic vulnerability? Is there such thing as a depression gene? In 2003, a study published in *Science* suggested that those with genetic variation in their serotonin transporter were three times more likely to be depressed.[26] But six years later this idea was wiped out by a meta-analysis of 14,000 patients published in the *Journal of the American Medical Association* that denied such an association.[27] Dr. Thomas Insel, director of the National Institute of Mental Health, commented with the following: "Despite high expectations, neither genomics nor imaging has yet impacted the diagnosis or treatment of the 45 million Americans with serious or moderate mental illness each year."[28] Dr. Carlat speaks the truth in his own words: "And where there is a scientific vacuum, drug companies are happy to insert a marketing message and call it science. As a result, psychiatry has become a proving ground for outrageous manipulations of science in the service of profit."[29]

Suffice it to say the data has poked so many holes in the serotonin theory that even the field of psychiatry itself is putting down its sword. In a 2005 essay for *PLOS Medicine* by Drs. Jeffrey R. Lacasse and Jonathan Leo, the authors gathered sentiments from influential thinkers in the field, including conventional clinicians and researchers who have expressed doubt on the entirety of what psychiatry has to offer around antidepressants (see tables on the following pages).[30]

The medical-pharmaceutical complex has constructed quite a few houses of cards, and far too many of its treatments—very profitable treatments—are offered without solid evidence to support doing so. In fact, only two studies are required for FDA licensure of most pharmaceuticals, essentially leaving the population to participate in a post-marketing experiment in which adverse effects—causalities—are monitored passively. It's a fabrication of science to think these drugs have a place in medicine, what is meant to be the art of healing. It could be argued that antidepressants are the new tobacco, and, like the tobacco industry, Big Pharma can wield a lot of power through clever marketing to seduce and influence us in stealthy, seemingly benign ways that are anything but.

DIRECT-TO-CONSUMER ADVERTISING

Sadly, direct-to-consumer advertising (DTCA) in America has allowed pharmaceutical companies to "teach" the public about brain chemical imbalances and serotonin deficiencies via sound bites

TABLE 1. EVIDENCE THE CHEMICAL IMBALANCE THEORY OF DEPRESSION IS NOT VALID: SELECTED QUOTATIONS

Quote	Citation
"By 1970…[biochemist and Nobel Prize Winner Julius] Axelrod had concluded that, whatever was wrong in depression, it was not lowered serotonin."	Healy, 2004, p. 12
"I spent the first several years of my career doing full-time research on brain serotonin metabolism, but I never saw any convincing research that any psychiatric disorder, including depression, results from a deficiency of brain serotonin" (Psychiatrist David Burns, who conducted award-winning serotonin research in the 1970s).	Lacasse & Gomory, 2003, p. 393
"Tianeptine is an interesting compound with antidepressant activity thought to be related to increased rather than decreased 5HT [serotonin] uptake" [meaning, in 1989 it was known to be an antidepressant that depletes, not increases, serotonin].	Ives & Heym, 1989, p. 22
"The simplistic idea of the '5-HT [serotonin]' neurone does not bear any relation to reality" (John Evenden, Astra pharmaceutical company research scientist, 1990).	Shorter, 2009, p. 204
"In the 1990s…No one knew if SSRIs raised or lowered serotonin levels; they still don't know…There was no evidence that treatment corrected anything."	Healy, 2015
"…Patients have been diagnosed with 'chemical imbalances' despite the fact that no test exists to support such a claim, and there is no real conception of what a correct chemical imbalance would look like…Yet conclusions such as 'depression is a biochemical imbalance' are created out of nothing more than semantics and the wishful thinking of scientists/psychiatrists and a public that will believe anything now that has the stamp of approval of medical science" (Psychiatrist David Kaiser of Northwestern University Hospital, 1996).	Kaiser, 1996; Lynch, 2015, pp. 31-32.
"Although it is often stated with great confidence that depressed people have a serotonin or norepinephrine deficiency, the evidence actually contradicts these claims" (Neuroscientist Elliot Valenstein).	Valenstein, 1998, p. 100
"The monamine hypothesis…holds that monoamines…such as… [serotonin]…are deficient in depression and that the action of antidepressants depends on increasing the synaptic availability of these monoamines….However, inferring neurotransmitter pathophysiology from…[SSRIs]…is similar to concluding that because aspirin causes gastrointestinal bleeding, headaches are caused by too much blood…Additional experience has not confirmed the monoamine depletion hypothesis." (American Psychiatric Association *Textbook of Psychiatry*, 1999).	Dubovsky & Buzan, 1999, p. 516
"A serotonin deficiency for depression has not been found" (Psychiatrist Joseph Glenmullen, Clinical Instructor of Psychiatry at Harvard Medical School).	Glenmullen, 2000, p. 197
"…I wrote that Prozac was no more, and perhaps less, effective in treating major depression than prior medications….I argued that the theories of brain functioning that led to the development of Prozac must be wrong or incomplete" (Brown University Psychiatrist Peter Kramer, author of *Listening to Prozac*).	Kramer, 2002
"[We must] abandon the simplistic hypotheses of there being either an abnormally high or abnormally low function of a given neurotransmitter" (Avrid Carlson, Nobel Prize winner for his work on the neurotransmitter dopamine, 2002).	CINP Meeting with the Nobels (2003); Shorter, 2009, p. 204
"Indeed, no abnormality of serotonin in depression has ever been demonstrated" (Psychiatrist and historian David Healy in 2004).	Healy, 2004, p. 12

"Antidepressants and the Chemical Imbalance Theory of Depression: A Reflection and Update on the Discourse," *Behavior Therapist* 38, no. 7 (October 2015): 206–213. Reprinted with permission.

TABLE 2. PROMOTION OF THE CHEMICAL IMBALANCE THEORY OF DEPRESSION AS VALID: SELECTED QUOTATIONS

Quote	Source	Citation
"Celexa helps to restore the brain's chemical balance by increasing the supply of a chemical messenger in the brain called serotonin."	Celexa website, 2005	Lacasse & Leo, 2005
"Antidepressants may be prescribed to correct imbalances in the levels of chemicals in the brain."	*Let's Talk Facts About Depression*, a patient information leaflet distributed by APA	American Psychiatric Association, 2005, p. 2
"Antidepressants…have no effect on normal mood. They restore brain chemistry to normal."	Nada Stotland, president of the American Psychiatric Association, 2007-2008	Stotland, 2001, p. 65
"[antidepressants work] only if there was a chemical imbalance in the brain that needed fixing"	Donald Klein, psychiatrist and psychopharmacologist	Talan, 1997
"While the patient may require a somatic therapy to correct the underlying chemical imbalance, he may also need psychotherapy…"	Nancy Andreason, psychiatrist and author of *The Broken Brain*	Andreason, 1985, p. 258
"…some depressed patients who have abnormally low levels of serotonin respond to SSRIs…"	Psychiatrist Richard Friedman in *The New York Times*	Friedman, 2007
"There is truly a real deficiency of serotonin in depressed patients."	Psychiatrist Charles Nemeroff	Nemeroff, 2007
"The physician should stress that depression is a highly treatable medical illness caused by a chemical imbalance."	MacArthur Foundation Depression Education Program for Primary Care Physicians	Cole, Raju, Barrett, Gerrity, & Dietrich, 2000, p. 340
"Patients with neurotransmitter dysregulation may have an imbalance of serotonin and norepinephrine…duloxetine [Cymbalta] may aid in correcting the imbalance of serotonin and norepinephrine neurotransmission in the brain."	Madkur Trivedi, psychiatrist at University of Texas Southwest Medical School, in The Primary Care Companion of the *Journal of Clinical Psychiatry*	Trivedi, 2004, p. 13
"Restoring serotonin's imbalances not only helps brighten mood and restore normal sleeping and eating patterns, but it also seems to promote a sense of well-being."	Michael Thase, psychiatrist and psychopharmacology researcher at the University of Pennsylvania, and science writer Susan Lang	Thase & Lang, 2004, p. 106
"We now know that mental illnesses—such as depression or schizophrenia—are not 'moral weaknesses' or imagined but real diseases caused by abnormalities of brain structure and imbalances in chemicals of the brain….medications and other treatments can correct these imbalances. Talk therapy can directly improve brain functioning."	Richard Harding, president of the American Psychiatric Association, 2000-2001	Harding, 2001, p. 66
"At some time in the course of their illness, most patients and families need some explanation of what has happened and why. Sometimes the explanation is as simplistic as 'a chemical imbalance'.…"	Robert Freedman, psychiatrist at the University of Colorado	Freedman, 2003, as cited by Hickey, 2014

and cleverly worded taglines that escape FDA policing. I have patients who come in believing that the solution is in a pill—what they've learned essentially from commercials. It's been calculated that DTCA advertising is responsible for nearly half (49 percent) of requests for drugs.[31] And fully seven out of ten times doctors prescribe based on appeals made by patients who learned through their computers and televisions that they have an "imbalance" that must be fixed with a pill.[32]

In the ten-year period between 1999 and 2008, DTCA tripled, from $1.3 to $4.8 billion, their efforts at educating patients about their need for psychiatric medication. The modern drug business has been built on "brain" medicines. Valium was the first blockbuster, selling 2 billion tablets in 1978. Then in the 1990s came Prozac, which defined the industry. The pharmaceutical industry spent $4.53 billion on direct-to-consumer advertising in the United States alone in 2014, up 18 percent from the previous year.[33]

The flagrant disconnect between the advertisements and scientific literature has been written about for more than a decade now, but you probably haven't read about it. It was clearly stated by Drs. Lacasse and Leo in their 2005 paper: "These advertisements present a seductive concept, and the fact that patients are now presenting with a self-described 'chemical imbalance' shows that the [advertising] is having its intended effect: the medical marketplace is being shaped in a way that is advantageous to the pharmaceutical companies."[34] As far back as 1998, at the dawn of consumer advertising of SSRIs, Professor Emeritus of Psychology and Neuroscience Elliot Valenstein of the University of Michigan summarized the scientific data by concluding, "What physicians and the public are reading about mental illness is by no means a neutral reflection of all the information that is available."[35]

The United States and New Zealand are the only countries in the world that allow advertisement on television for prescription drugs. In 1997, a change to an FDA regulation opened the floodgates on direct-to-consumer advertising, allowing drug makers to promote their wares on television. This also paved the way for celebrities, athletes, models, and aging baby boomers to dominate those ads.

Given these forces, along with the number of symptoms listed under antidepressant use, it's really no surprise that more than $11 billion is spent each year on these medications.[36] Pharmaceutical companies have more than six hundred lobbyists, and they finance more than 70 percent of FDA trials.[37] They court physicians, toss them copious free samples, pay consultants to speak at scientific meetings, advertise in medical journals, fund medical education, and ghostwrite, selectively choosing and redundantly submitting data for publication. Psychiatric studies funded by Big Pharma are four times more likely to be published if they report positive results. Only 18 percent of psychiatrists disclose their conflicts of interest when they publish data.[38] Their studies allow for all kinds of indiscretions, such as removing people who are likely to respond to placebo before the study to strengthen the perceived benefit and using sedative medications with the study's medications, thereby skewing results in favor of the drug (more on this shortly).

A now famous 2008 study in the *New England Journal of Medicine* led by Dr. Erick Turner at Portland VA Medical Centers sought to expose the extent of data manipulation.[39] Through valiant efforts to uncover unpublished data, he and his team determined that from 1987 to 2004, twelve antidepressants were approved based on seventy-four studies; thirty-eight were positive, and thirty-seven of these were published. Thirty-six were negative (showing no benefit), and three of these were published as such, while eleven were published with a positive spin (always read the data, not the author's conclusion!), and twenty-two were unpublished.

The FDA requires only two studies for drug approval, so you can see how these companies are tossing the coin over and over again until heads comes up and hoping no one is looking when it's tails. To get a sense of just how misleading the pharmaceutical industry can be, consider the largest study to date funded by the National Institute of Mental Health, conducted at the University of Texas in 2006.[40] It cost the public $35 million for researchers to follow more than four thousand patients who were treated with Celexa over twelve months. This was not a double-blind placebo controlled study, so the people knew what they were getting. Half of them reportedly improved at eight weeks. Those who didn't were switched to Wellbutrin, Effexor, or Zoloft or "augmented" with Buspar or Wellbutrin. Guess what? It didn't matter who took what, because the same percentage of the group allegedly improved (18 to 30 percent) no matter what drug they were on. Only 3 percent of patients were supposedly in remission at twelve months. Now here's where the story gets interesting.

In February 2012, a suit was filed against Celexa's maker, Forest Pharmaceuticals, alleging that the company paid a bribe to the principal investigator of this particular study to fix the results in favor of Celexa.[41] The suit was settled out of court, and it came on the heels of the company having to pay a criminal fine of $150 million and forfeit assets of $14 million for suppressing and misrepresenting data on the negative effects of using their drug to treat adolescents. Celexa was only approved to treat adults, but in pursuit of selling more drugs and increasing profits, the company targeted doctors who treated children and teens.[42]

It's a foregone conclusion: these practices sabotage the accuracy of data and convey information that corrupts a doctor's delivery of care and endangers patients. The tragic cost of this data manipulation is the loss of true informed consent. Physicians cannot adequately share with their patients the risks and benefits if the benefits are fabricated and the risks are not uncovered or are unacknowledged. What's more, these drugs are no more effective than a placebo. As far back as 1984, the National Institute of Mental Health was quoted as saying: "Elevations or decrements in the functioning of serotonergic systems per se are not likely to be associated with depression." The good old placebo effect likely explains any perceived short-term effects from the antidepressants.

SHORT-TERM EFFICACY:
THE POWER OF THE PLACEBO EFFECT

Despite Big Pharma's efforts, the truth about these brain bombs is emerging. In 1998, the year direct-to-consumer advertising took off, Harvard psychologist and researcher Dr. Irving Kirsch, an established and respected expert on the placebo effect, published a landmark meta-analysis of nearly three thousand patients who were treated with antidepressants, psychotherapy, placebo, or no treatment.[43] The results of the study became front-page news and received widespread attention—and criticism. Kirsch found that placebo duplicated 75 percent of the drug's effect, that non-antidepressant medications had the same effect as antidepressants, and that the remaining 25 percent of the apparent drug effect was attributable to what's called the "active placebo effect."

Kirsch uses this term to refer to the effect of the mere *belief* in antidepressants—a belief that is triggered by the experience of side effects such as nausea, headache, and dry mouth. What happens in a trial is that subjects are put in either the placebo group or the medication group without knowing which group they were assigned to. Because the placebo is without side effects (an inactive placebo), when they develop side effects, all of those commercial-inspired beliefs about their brain's chemical correction are kicked into high gear, and at least a quarter of these people begin feeling better because of it.

So how much can we thank the placebo effect when we experience fewer symptoms while taking an antidepressant? The backlash to Kirsch's study inspired him to continue exploring the power of the placebo. By 2008 he'd published another compelling meta-analysis study that further stirred up an incendiary response from critics.[44] This time he leveraged the Freedom of Information Act to access unpublished studies and found that when these unpublished studies were included, antidepressants outperformed placebo in only twenty of forty-six trials. That's less than half! What's more, the overall difference between drugs and placebos was 1.7 points on the 52-point Hamilton Rating Scale for Depression, used to rate depression in clinical research. Put simply, this small increment is clinically insignificant, and likely accounted for by minor side effects (such as activation and sedation).

The response to this publication led Kirsch to come out with another paper that clearly laid out the facts, counterchallenged his critics, and further demonstrated the power of the placebo.[45] In his concluding thoughts, he writes: "Without accurate knowledge, patients and physicians cannot make informed treatment decisions, researchers will be asking the wrong questions, and policymakers will be implementing misinformed policies. If the antidepressant effect is largely a placebo effect, it is important that we know this. It means that improvement can be obtained without reliance on addictive drugs with potentially serious side effects."

When Kirsch's book *The Emperor's New Drugs: Exploding the Antidepressant Myth* came out in 2010 with proof that antidepressants do not have a clinically meaningful advantage over placebo, his analysis was acknowledged by researchers as a valid albeit provocative contribution to medical literature. But it didn't change clinical psychiatry or the number of antidepressants prescribed, and it continued to incur the criticism and even rage of prescribing psychiatrists desperate to pick apart his findings to defend their now baseless practices. It's hard to blame them—they put a lot of time, money, and effort into learning mistruths around antidepressants! The irony in Kirsch's findings is that the results came from studies that were underwritten and designed *by the drug companies themselves*. These studies were conducted in a way that would give the drugs an advantage, yet they still didn't outperform the placebo.[46]

In order for a drug to be approved, it must be shown to be superior to placebo. As you can imagine, drug companies despise placebo effects. They will do everything in their power to minimize the impact of placebo in their studies. That the FDA allows them to use these techniques is wrong, another example of Big Pharma's shameless misconduct.

Because the FDA database contains all of the data from initial trials, both published and unpublished, analyzing its data is exceptionally useful. Keep in mind that drug companies normally don't publish negative results. They prefer to file away those studies in a drawer where they will never be found; hence the "file drawer" phenomenon.

A fascinating 2014 study published in the *Journal of Clinical Psychiatry*, one of my field's most respected journals, explored—and exposed—the real power of belief in psychiatric treatment. A group of researchers at Columbia University analyzed data from two large, multicenter discontinuation trials encompassing 673 people diagnosed with major depressive disorder and who were taking fluoxetine (generic Prozac) for twelve weeks.[47] After those three months, they were told that they'd be randomized to either a placebo or continued fluoxetine. So while they all knew they were taking the antidepressant in the first three months, they didn't know if what they were given afterward was an active antidepressant or a sugar pill. The results spoke for themselves: both groups—the ones still taking the fluoxetine and those on the placebo—experienced a *worsening* of depressive symptoms. This outcome suggests two significant interpretations: (1) the initial effect during the first three months was attributable to placebo, as all patients knew they were receiving treatment; and (2) the worsening of symptoms upon the mere possibility of getting just a placebo is indicative of the *undoing of the placebo effect*, what's sometimes called the *nocebo* effect.

Identifying a tremendous placebo effect has been further echoed by other meta-analyses. The power of belief and the expectation of healing cannot be dismissed when medical treatments appear to work. In my opinion, the use of medications associated with serious short- and long-term side effects and which primarily ride the placebo effect represents an ethically questionable practice.

I work with the placebo effect every day in my office because I aim to inspire a different set of beliefs. Even people who claim to be suicidal can experience the placebo effect under my care. The decision to consider taking your own life is not a trait that would have been selected for over the millennia of human evolution. It's more logical to assume it has roots in physiological imbalances, which is where I like to spend my time searching for solutions with my patients. I look for problems like nutrient deficiencies, endocrine disruption, and autoimmunity. The first and most important thing I like to convey to patients is that they are in charge. They have agency. This sensibility can go a long way, because they're coming to me thinking I have what they don't have—a quick fix. A quick fix is a lovely idea, and if one existed, it could be great. Unfortunately, the weight of the data suggests that it doesn't and that we may be doing more harm than good by collectively pretending it does. The challenge is that it's human nature to feel better after doing something we *think* will make us feel better. But sometimes inaction is the best medicine.

LONG-TERM SIDE EFFECTS: MORE MEDS, MORE DEPRESSION, MORE DISABILITY . . . AND DEATH?

But you might ask, "What if these drugs are in fact working some of the time for some people?" They still wouldn't be worth the consequences for the placebo effect, particularly given their side effects, which are notoriously hidden from the lay public. I find it outrageous that drug companies can use any number of tactics to establish efficacy, including the suppression of data, and then use those tactics to legitimize long-term prescribing with no thought or attention to the real side effects over time.

When I lecture on the futility and perils of antidepressants, I like to employ the following analogy courtesy of Dr. David Healy, an internationally respected psychiatrist based in the UK: Let's say you're somebody who experiences a lot of social anxiety. You have a couple glasses of wine at a party as a preemptive strike. A sense of calmness washes over you and your symptoms evaporate. Through deductive reasoning, you could say, "Well, I must have an alcohol deficiency, so I should continue to consume alcohol every time I have this symptom, and I might want to drink regularly to prevent it altogether." This analogy is emblematic of the practice of dishing out antidepressants without any consideration of their long-term consequences.[48]

We've arrived at a place in psychiatry's abuse of antidepressants where we have a half-baked theory in a vacuum of science that the pharmaceutical industry raced to fill. We have the illusion of short-term efficacy and assumptions about long-term safety. The potential emerging side effects are nothing short of horrifying, from suppressed libido and sexual dysfunction, abnormal bleeding, insomnia, migraine, weight gain, and blood sugar imbalances to risk of violent, irrational behavior and suicide. Before I get to the ugliest of side effects and withdrawal complications, let's focus on how your ability to function long term in the world with depression is significantly sabotaged by treating that first episode of depression with medication. This too has been expertly explored by Robert Whitaker, whose website (www.madinamerica.com) is a virtual library of published data and thoughtful reviews of multiple long-term studies that have followed large groups of people taking antidepressants. Time and time again these studies demonstrate poor functional outcomes for people treated with antidepressants relative to those with minimal to no medication treatment.[49] They are at greater risk for all the acute side effects I've already listed, as well as increased risk of relapse, cognitive impairment, secondary diagnosis and medication treatments (first a depression diagnosis followed by a bipolar one), and recurrent hospitalization.

A breathtaking 60 percent of patients are still diagnosed with depression one year into treatment, despite temporary improvement within the first three months.[50] Two prospective studies in particular support a *worse* outcome in those prescribed medication. In one such British study, an unmedicated group experienced a 62 percent improvement by six months, whereas the drug-treated patients experienced only a 33 percent reduction in symptoms.[51] And in another study of depressed patients conducted by the World Health

Organization (WHO) in fifteen cities across the UK, it was found that at the end of one year, those who weren't exposed to psychotropic medications enjoyed much better "general health," their depressive symptoms were much "milder," and they were less likely to still be "mentally ill"![52]

Now let's consider the more serious possible side effects of violent behavior, relapse, and crippling withdrawal among those who try to escape their grip. Antidepressants have a well-established history of causing violent side effects, including suicide and homicide. In fact, five of the top ten most violence-inducing drugs have been found to be antidepressants.[53] Over the past three decades there have been hundreds of mass shootings, murders, and other violent episodes that have been committed by individuals on psychiatric drugs. Big Pharma spends around $2.4 billion a year on their direct-to-consumer television advertising for drugs like Zoloft, Prozac, and Paxil. The networks can't afford to run negative stories about prescription drugs, as they would lose tens of millions of dollars in ad revenue (no wonder the connection is habitually downplayed or ignored entirely). The Russian roulette of patients vulnerable to these "side effects" is only beginning to be known and may have something to do with how their bodies (and actions of their unique genetic code) metabolize these chemicals and preexisting allostatic (stress) load. Dr. Healy has worked tirelessly to expose data implicating antidepressants in risk of suicide and violence, maintaining a database for reporting, writing, and lecturing about cases of medication-induced death that could make your soul wince. And what about our most vulnerable: new mothers of helpless infants? I have countless patients like Kate in my practice who report never-before thoughts of suicide within weeks of starting an antidepressant for postpartum depression.

In a population where only a few randomized trials have examined the use of antidepressants for postpartum depression, I have grave concerns for women who are treated with drugs before more benign and effective interventions such as dietary modification, thyroid treatment, and addressing their sleep habits during this period when sleep deprivation runs high are explored. We already know that "low mood" is likely to resolve on its own within three months without any treatment, and upward of 70 percent of people will be free of depression without any medication whatsoever within a year.[54] Yet we reflexively turn to these drugs and their unpredictable effects that can rob us of the ability to find permanent relief through the body's own powerful systems, even though, by their own claims, they take six to eight weeks to "take effect."

In 2004, the U.S. Food and Drug Administration (FDA) revised the labeling requirements for antidepressant medications with a warning that: "Antidepressants increased the risk compared to placebo of suicidal thinking and behavior (suicidality) in children, adolescents, and young adults in short-term studies of major depressive disorder (MDD) and other psychiatric disorders."[55] The FDA was pushed to revise the labeling following a bevy of lawsuits in which pharmaceutical companies were forced to reveal previously undisclosed drug data.

You'd think such labeling would give people—and parents—pause. But since 2004, antidepressant use has only increased among both children and adults. I am routinely helping women who want to have a baby either avoid or taper from antidepressants, despite having been "specially trained" to prescribe for this population. For many of them, the first step is simply accepting the fact that they've been lied to about the value of antidepressants and their alleged benefits. Meanwhile, their downsides are not only downplayed but actively concealed.

All you have to do is spend a few minutes on SurvivingAntidepressants.org, BeyondMeds.com, or SSRIstories.org to appreciate that we have created a monster. Millions of men, women, and children the world over are suffering side effects, including complicated withdrawal routinely dismissed by their prescribing clinicians. Contrary to what Big Pharma would have you believe, weaning off antidepressants is extremely difficult, so choosing to take them could be signing up for a lifetime of medication use that creates and sustains abnormal states in the brain and entire nervous system. As a clinician who once believed in these medications, I have been humbled by what they are capable of. In fact, even when I have tapered women off of Celexa at extremely low increments of .001 mg a month, it can be hard to imagine another class of substances on earth so potentially complicated to discontinue.

I first became aware of the habit-forming nature of these medications when I worked with a patient who wanted to become pregnant in the coming year to taper off of Zoloft. She experienced about six months of protracted withdrawal that began at about two months after her last dose. My training did nothing to prepare me to deal with that.

The truth is that we have very little idea about what these medications are actually doing! At the same time, though, we need to acknowledge that the complexity of neurophysiology is overwhelming. Although the appeal is to think that we've cracked the code on human behavior and all of its intricate physiology, we're far from it. For example, ten years ago we didn't even know that the brain had an immune system, and two years ago we didn't know it had lymphatics—basic anatomy. We used to think that immune activity in the brain only happened under certain pathological circumstances. But now we've identified microglia—billions of cells that play a specific role in managing inflammatory responses in the brain based on perceived threats from the rest of the body.[56] And it's not just about tinkering with chemical levels in the brain or the body for that matter.

We like to cling to simple explanations, but even the categorical name of the various antidepressants, *selective serotonin reuptake inhibitors,* is misleading. They are far from selective. In September 2014, an alarming new study from the Max Planck Institute in Leipzig, Germany, showed that even *a single dose* of an antidepressant can alter the brain's architecture *within three hours,* changing the brain's functional connectivity.[57] The study, published in the journal *Current Biology,* was shocking not only to the health journalists who reported on it, but also to the doctors who prescribe these drugs.

An important analysis by the former director of the NIMH and published in the *American Journal of Psychiatry* shows that antidepressants "create perturbations in neurotransmitter functions," causing the body to adapt through a series of biological events that occur after "chronic administration," leading to brains that after a few weeks function in a way that is "qualitatively as well as quantitatively different from the normal state."[58] In other words, the brain's natural functionality is assaulted by the medication to the point that it can become permanent. That said, everything we will explore in this book speaks to the body's tremendous and almost unstoppable resilience when properly supported.

Dr. Paul Andrews of the Virginia Institute for Psychiatric and Behavioral Genetics demonstrated through a careful meta-analysis of forty-six studies that a patient's risk of relapse is directly proportionate to how disruptive the medication is to the brain.[59] The more disruptive the medication, the higher the risk of relapse upon discontinuation. He and his colleagues challenge the whole notion of relapse, suggesting that when you feel terrible upon stopping an antidepressant, what you're experiencing is *withdrawal*—not a return of your mental illness. And when you choose the medication route, you're actually extending the duration of your depression. Andrews writes: ". . . unmedicated patients have much shorter episodes, and better long-term prospects, than medicated patients . . . [T]he average duration of an untreated episode of major depression is twelve to thirteen weeks."[60]

In a retrospective ten-year study in the Netherlands, 76 percent of those with unmedicated depression recovered without relapse relative to 50 percent of those treated.[61] Unlike the mess of contradictory studies around short-term effects, there are no comparable studies that show a better outcome in those prescribed antidepressants long term.

Harvard researchers have also concluded that at least 50 percent of drug-withdrawn patients relapsed within fourteen months.[62] In the words of one team of researchers led by Dr. Rif El-Mallakh from the University of Louisville: "[L]ong-term antidepressant use may be depressogenic . . . it is possible that antidepressant agents modify the hardwiring of neuronal synapses [which] not only render antidepressants ineffective but also induce a resident, refractory depressive state." Dr. El-Mallakh and his colleagues wrote this bold statement in a letter to the editor of the *Journal of Clinical Psychiatry* in 1999.[63] Then, in 2011, they published a new paper including eighty-five citations proving that antidepressants make things worse in the long run.[64] (So when your doctor says, "You see, look how sick you are, you shouldn't have stopped that medication," you should know that the data suggests that your symptoms are signs of withdrawal, not relapse.)

In *Anatomy of an Epidemic,* Robert Whitaker summarizes the matter succinctly:

> We can now see how the antidepressant story all fits together, and why the widespread use of these drugs would contribute to a rise in the number of disabled mentally ill in the United States. Over the short term, those who take an antidepressant will likely see their symptoms lessen. They will see this as proof that the drugs work, as will their doctors. However, this short-term amelioration of symptoms is not markedly greater than what is seen in patients treated with a placebo, and this initial use also puts them onto a problematic long-term course. If they stop taking the medications, they are at high risk of relapsing. But if they stay on the drugs, they will also likely suffer recurrent episodes of depression, and this chronicity increases the risk that they will become disabled. The SSRIs, to a certain extent, act like a trap in the same way that neuroleptics [tranquilizers] do.[65]

More than twenty years have passed since clinicians and researchers started collecting evidence against antidepressants. Although these drugs may offer relief in the short term thanks to the placebo effect, they lead to chronic, persistent depression that resists treatment when taken for an extended period of time. In some people, stopping the drug can cause a slow and gradual lightening of the mood, but this doesn't always occur, and depression can become more or less permanent. Remember the alcohol effect.

Not surprisingly, the powers that be in my field have not looked into this matter or launched a serious investigation. And yet the studies keep emerging. In early 2015, yet another headline hit that Big Pharma turned a blind eye to. It read "Stopping SSRI Antidepressants Can Cause Long, Intense Withdrawal Problems" and referred to the first systematic review of withdrawal problems that patients experience when trying to get off SSRI antidepressant medications.[66] A team of American and Italian researchers found that withdrawing from SSRIs was in many ways comparable to trying to quit addictive benzodiazepine sedatives and barbiturates.[67] They also discovered that withdrawal symptoms aren't fleeting; they can last months or even years. Moreover, entirely new, persistent psychiatric disorders can surface from discontinuing SSRIs.

The authors analyzed fifteen randomized controlled studies, four open trials, four retrospective investigations, and thirty-eight case reports of SSRI withdrawal. Paroxetine (Paxil) was found to be the worst, but all the SSRI antidepressants were documented as causing a wide range of withdrawal symptoms from dizziness, electrical shock sensations, and diarrhea to anxiety, panic, agitation, insomnia, and severe depression. They write: "Symptoms typically occur within a few days from drug discontinuation and last a few weeks, also with gradual tapering. However, many variations are possible, including late onset and/or longer persistence of disturbances. Symptoms may be easily misidentified as signs of impending relapse."

In their conclusions, they state what should be the obvious: "Clinicians need to add SSRIs to the list of drugs potentially inducing withdrawal symptoms upon discontinuation, together with benzodiazepines, barbiturates, and other psychotropic drugs." An accompanying editorial to their paper notes that "This type of withdrawal consists of: (1) the return of the original illness at a greater intensity and/or with additional features of the illness, and/or (2) symptoms related to emerging new disorders. They persist at least six weeks after drug withdrawal and are sufficiently severe and disabling to have patients return to their previous drug treatment. When the previous drug treatment is not restarted, post-withdrawal disorders may last for several months to years."

The editorial also states that "With SSRI withdrawal, persistent postwithdrawal disorders may appear as new psychiatric disorders, in particular disorders that can be treated successfully with SSRIs and SNRIs. Significant postwithdrawal illnesses found with SSRI use include anxiety disorders, tardive insomnia, major depression, and bipolar illness."

This bit of news is extremely unsettling to current practices in psychiatry. According to the current American Psychological Association treatment guidelines for major depressive disorder, "During the maintenance phase, an antidepressant medication that produced symptom remission during the acute phase and maintained remission during the continuation phase should be continued at a full therapeutic dose." Such a guideline merely promotes more drug sales, and more crippling side effects.

DON'T GO DOWN THE RABBIT HOLE

We need to break out of the spell that the pharmaceutical industry has put us under. Psychiatry's swan song has been sung; listen for its plaintive wail. We must reject the serotonin meme and start looking at depression (and anxiety, and bipolar disorder, and schizophrenia, and OCD) for what they are: disparate expressions of a body struggling to adapt to a stressor. There are times in our evolution as a cultural species that we need to unlearn what we know and change what we think is true. We have to move out of the comfort of certainty and into the freeing light of uncertainty. It is from this space of acknowledged unknowing that we can truly grow.[68]

From my vantage point, this growth will encompass a sense of wonder—both a curiosity about what symptoms of mental illness may be telling us about our physiology and spirit and a sense of humbled awe at all that we do not yet have the tools to appreciate. For this reason, honoring our coevolution with the natural world and sending the body a signal of safety through movement, diet, meditation, and environmental detoxification represents our most primal and most powerful tool for healing. We also need to identify vulnerabilities and chemical exposures and support basic cellular function, detoxification, and immune response. This is, ultimately, personalized medicine.

To me, the worst part of the misguided mess we've made of mental health care is that we are missing out on the potential for true resilience and self-healing. Safe, effective alternatives to help us through these passages in life do indeed exist. Perhaps most concerning to a holistic physician is data that suggests that long-term antidepressant treatment actually compromises the benefits of exercise![69] The effects of exercise have been shown to be comparable to Zoloft but can be diminished when combined with Zoloft; patients relapse at higher rates than they do with exercise alone. I'll be going into much greater detail about exercise in Chapter 7, and I'll share why I think this is the case. Exercise is an antidote to depression best used without antidepressants.

Mental health will always be grounded in whole body health. When you discover the real imbalances underlying all your symptoms—physical and mental—and take steps to address them, you can restore your health without resorting to problematic drug treatments and endless psychotherapy.

The next question to answer is: What kind of "imbalances" come under the veil of depression? We'll find out in the next chapter.

CHAPTER 3

The New Biology of Depression

What Gut Microbes and Silent Inflammation
Have to Do with Mental Health

Depression is often an inflammation-driven condition, not a
neurochemical deficiency disease.

The most powerful path to our brain—and peace of mind—is
through our gut.

Pick up any health or diet book published recently and you'll
likely read about the ills of chronic inflammation and the
blessings of the human microbiome. The two have been the science
buzzwords of late, and for good reason. These concepts reflect the
zeitgeist of the modern patient because we have reached a point
in our collective evolution where our health is being outpaced by
lifestyles that are not aligned with how we are biologically designed
to live. We are idle when our bodies want to move, we eat foods
that are unrecognizable to our systems, and we expose ourselves to
environmental factors that assault our cells. This incompatibility
is creating serious internal conflict and driving rampant levels of
chronic inflammation like an alarm that won't shut off.

Inflammation is often described as underlying virtually every
chronic condition and illness, from obesity, heart disease, and diabetes to degenerative illnesses including dementia and cancer. I've

already mentioned inflammation dozens of times already, because science is telling us that depression is also an inflammatory condition. In this model, depression is a general fever that tells us little about what is actually causing the body to react and protect itself in this way. The body is "hot," and we need to understand why. Depressive symptoms are merely the manifestation of many downstream effects on hormones and neurotransmitters, but if we were to swim up to the source, we would find a river of inflammatory markers coursing by. The source itself may be a single culprit, such as a dietary ingredient to which the body adversely reacts or a collection of culprits that have indirect effects on the internal workings of the brain because of their impact on the immune system and stress response. In fact, the relationship between depression and inflammation is so compelling that researchers are now exploring the use of immune-altering medications to treat depression.[1]

Researchers are desperately searching for the next frontier because the current model is in crisis. As you have seen, modern psychiatry has served as a repository for the diagnostic and therapeutic limitations of conventional medicine. When a patient's symptoms of malaise, "brain fog," lethargy, inattention, insomnia, agitation, and flat mood slip through the cracks of the discrete territories of specialty medicine, the patient is referred for psychiatric treatment. When she is treated with nonsteroidal anti-inflammatory drugs (NSAIDs), statins, acid blockers, antibiotics, and birth control pills, the effects of these medications are poorly grasped by prescribers, complaints are dismissed, and she is again referred for psychiatric care. What happens when psychiatric care itself is predicated on medication treatment, with placebo-driven short-term effects and worse functional outcomes in the long term? Perhaps it is time to acknowledge the failures of this paradigm.

Now that the scientific literature has demolished the serotonin model of depression, it can no longer stand on its own, and throwing more and more medications at a perceived false target is doing more harm than good. It's fitting that psychiatry would follow the investigative path of other chronic diseases such as arthritis, asthma, certain cancers, diabetes, autoimmunity, Alzheimer's disease, and heart disease—all of which can be the result of lifestyle barbs that drive inflammation.

Today the concept of psychoneuroimmunology has supplanted the myopic serotonin premise in the primary literature.[2,3] This new model reveals the interconnectedness of multiple systems—the gut, brain, and immune systems—and takes us out of a one-gene, one-ill, one-pill narrow perspective. The field of psychiatry has known about the role of the immune system in the onset of depression for nearly one hundred years. But only recently, thanks to better technology and large, long-term studies that reveal the impact of the relationship between immunity, inflammation, gut flora, and mental health, have we really begun to understand the relevant connections.[4]

Given our new awareness of the complexity of these connections, including the role of the microbiome, biology as we know it must come under revision, especially when applied to its direct human application in medical interventions. No longer can we say "she was born with it"—the dismissive meme that dominated a large part of twentieth-century medicine. Nor can we say that the same exposure causes the same illness in all people. According to conventional medicine, different genetic problems or infectious exposures cause different diseases for which there are distinct, one-pill solutions. And out of that "broken and vulnerable body" theory came the "me versus the microbial world" mentality. René Dubos, the famous microbiologist and early pioneer in the developmental origins of health and disease as well as the one to develop the first clinically tested antibiotic, warned us of the dangers of classical germ theory half a century ago:

[M]an himself has emerged from a line descent that began with microbial life, a line common to all plant and animal species . . . [he] is dependent not only on other human beings and on the physical world but also on other creatures— animals, plants, microbes—that have evolved together with him. Man will ultimately destroy himself if he thoughtlessly eliminates the organisms that constitute essential links in the complex and delicate web of life of which he is a part.[5]

Awareness of the role of microbes in our day-to-day life has brought us to a radical new understanding of the indelible fusions between the functions of the gut and brain. In fact, the role of the brain-based immune system has only been elucidated in the past ten years, and while many questions remain, the facts are swiftly building up to make an incontrovertible case against pharmaceuticals and for wholly natural approaches to wellness. In the words of Drs. Paula Garay and A. Kimberly McAllister of UC Davis, who address so-called immune molecules (the cells and their substances that respond to internal and external threats):

> . . . the sheer number of immune molecules that could be important for nervous system development and function is staggering. Although much progress has been made in the past 10 years in our appreciation that immune molecules play critical roles in the healthy brain, the large majority of immune molecules have not yet been studied for their presence and function in the brain. For the immune molecules that we know are important, almost nothing is understood about their mechanisms of action.[6]

Why hasn't this message made it to those who still believe we can safely manipulate human behavior through psychotropic drugs or that we shouldn't be concerned about the effects of immune-disrupting substances in our environment, from ingredients in foods to vaccines? Drug products were developed without even basic knowledge of this relevant physiology, let alone the implications for the role of the immune system in neurology. Only recently have scientists begun to look at how certain antipsychotics, including antidepressants, change the native tribes of bacteria in the body and render patients vulnerable to other health conditions. The drug desipramine, for example, has been shown to alter the composition of microbes in the mouth, causing dry mouth and gingivitis. Another example: olanzapine changes the microbial balance with results including metabolic injury and weight gain—especially in women. Remember, not until 2015 did we even know that the brain has a lymphatic system with a primary purpose of connecting it to the immune system. As the authors of that 2015 *Nature* paper stated: "The discovery of the central nervous system lymphatic system may call for a reassessment of basic assumptions in neuroimmunology and sheds new light on the aetiology of neuroinflammatory and neurodegenerative diseases associated with immune system dysfunction."[7]

It's time for that reassessment. It's time for disciplines like psychoneuroimmunology to take shape and provide a more accurate context for our understanding—those that honor the known and unknown complexities of the human organism in its environment.

So with all that in mind, let's deconstruct what is known about depression as it relates to inflammation and the gut-brain dance. I'll start with some basics about inflammation.

THE INFLAMMATORY MODEL OF DEPRESSION

As we all know, the immune system is essential to human health and well-being. It helps coordinate the body's response to its environment, from chemicals and medications to physical injuries and infections, essentially maintaining the critical divide between what is "self" and what is "other." At the heart of a healthy immune system is an ability to experience appropriate forms of inflammation, which I'll assume you're familiar with from a rudimentary level—the inflammation, for example, that accompanies a paper cut or sprained ankle. These reflect inflammatory responses we can actually feel and sometimes see (such as redness, swelling, and bruising). In this instance, inflammation is part of a necessary biological cascade enabling the body to defend itself against something it believes to be potentially harmful, and subsequently recalibrate.

When the trigger for inflammation becomes chronic, the effects can be directly toxic to our cells. Unlike the inflammation that follows bruising your arm or skinning your knee, this more silent, ongoing inflammation deep inside has a meaningful connection to your mental health.

The brain lacks pain receptors, so when we're showing signs of depression we can't feel inflammation in the brain like we do in a laceration or arthritic hip. Nonetheless, scientific research has clearly demonstrated over and over again that inflammation underlies the development of depression (and most other chronic diseases).

Several messengers relay information about inflammation between the brain and the body. A variety of inflammatory markers—chemical messengers called cytokines that tell us inflammation is occurring—are elevated in those with depression. These include markers like C-reactive protein and cytokines such as interleukins one and six (IL-1 and IL-6) and tumor necrosis factor alpha (TNF-α). Elevated cytokines in the blood have not only been shown to relate directly to a diagnosis of depression, but they are *predictive* of depression. In other words, the inflammation may be the trigger of rather than the response to depression.[8,9,10] As I briefly mentioned in Chapter 1, one of the most predictable side effects of interferon therapy for hepatitis C is depression. In fact, 45 percent of patients develop depression with interferon treatment, which appears to be related to elevated levels of inflammatory cytokines IL-6 and TNF.[11] But there's also compelling literature suggesting that even stress, specifically psychosocial stress, can cause this inflammation by mobilizing immature immune cells called macrophages from your bone marrow to start the inflammatory process.[12] So you can see how inflammation lies at the heart of a vicious cycle; the process can trigger depression just as it can be aggravated by depression.

Researchers have further found that in melancholic depression, bipolar disorder, and postpartum depression, white blood cells called monocytes turn on pro-inflammatory genes that lead to the release of cytokines, while leading to decreased cortisol sensitivity.[13]

Cortisol, you'll recall, is the body's chief stress hormone; it's also a buffer against inflammation. When your cells lose their sensitivity to cortisol, they become resistant to cortisol's message, and the result is prolonged inflammatory states. It helps to keep in mind that broadly speaking, the stress response largely dictates the inflammatory response and its perpetuation.

Once triggered in the body, the inflammatory agents transfer information to the central nervous system, typically through stimulation of major nerves such as the vagus, which connects the gut and brain (more on this shortly). Specialized cells in the brain called microglia represent the brain's immune hubs and are activated in inflammatory states. In activated microglia, an enzyme called IDO (indoleamine 2, 3-dioxygenase) stimulates the production of biomolecules that can result in symptoms such as anxiety and agitation. These are just some of the changes that may conspire to let your brain in on what your body may know is wrong.

Researchers have also observed that people with higher levels of these inflammatory markers are more likely to respond to anti-inflammatories than to antidepressants; this helps explain why curcumin (the golden-colored antioxidant in turmeric), a powerful anti-inflammatory made by nature, has been found to be superior to Prozac and especially effective when medication isn't.[14,15]

One of the most important takeaways from the new information gained about the role of inflammation in depression, in particular a continuous state of low-grade inflammation and the stress signals associated with it, is that in many cases it tends to be generated from an unlikely source: the gut. In millions of people today, the gut is largely disrupted due to something called intestinal dysbiosis. Let me explain.

LEAKY GUTS FANNING THE FLAMES OF INFLAMMATION AND DEPRESSION

First, some basic anatomy. Your gastrointestinal tract, the tube that goes from your esophagus to your anus, is lined with a single layer of epithelial cells. It's the largest mucosal surface, and this intestinal lining has three main functions. It's the means through which you obtain nutrients from the foods you eat. It prevents potentially harmful particles, chemicals, and organisms from getting into your bloodstream. And it's the home to specialized cells that patrol and present to the immune system suspected invaders. The immune system provides chemicals called immunoglobulins that bind to foreign proteins to protect the body from them.

The body uses two pathways to absorb nutrients from the gut. One moves nutrients *through* the epithelial cells (transcellular); the other moves nutrients *between* the epithelial cells (paracellular). The connections between cells are called tight junctions, and as you can imagine, each of these complex, exceedingly small intersections is regulated. If they somehow become compromised and overly permeable, a condition called "leaky gut" develops. And because these junctions act as gatekeepers—keeping potential threats that will provoke the immune system out—they greatly influence levels of inflammation. We in the medical community now know that when your intestinal barrier is damaged, a spectrum of health challenges can result, not the least of which is depression.

What happens is that when these tight junctions are compromised, undigested food particles, cell debris, and bacteria components can sneak by to stir trouble in the bloodstream with downstream effects that manifest in depressive symptoms. To quote one team of researchers from Belgium: "There is now evidence that major depression (MDD) is accompanied by an activation of the inflammatory response system and that pro-inflammatory cytokines and lipopolysaccharide (LPS) may induce depressive symptoms."[16] Later on, we'll see how ingredients like gluten, sugar and artificial sweeteners, casein proteins (dairy), and processed vegetable oils can activate the immune system and result in pro-inflammatory cytokines coursing through your system. But let's look at what LPS alone could be doing. This is an interesting area of study just coming into view.

THE LPS BOMB

Lipopolysaccharide (LPS) is not only a mouthful of a word, but it's among the most villainous of biological threats. It flips on inflammatory pathways in the body like a switch. LPS is a combination of lipids (fat) and sugars, and is found on the outer membrane of certain bacteria that are naturally found in the gut, representing as much as 50 to 70 percent of the intestinal flora. LPS serves to protect these bacteria so they are not digested by bile salts from the gallbladder. LPS is not supposed to travel beyond the interior of the gut, however, but it can if the gut lining is somehow compromised.

LPS induces a violent inflammatory response in humans—so violent that it's also termed *endotoxin*, meaning a toxin that comes from within.[17] It's used experimentally in laboratory research to instantly create inflammation in animal models to study the full array of illnesses rooted in inflammation, from inflammatory bowel disorders, diabetes, lupus, rheumatoid arthritis, and multiple sclerosis to depression, Parkinson's disease, Alzheimer's disease, and even autism. In a healthy individual whose intestinal lining is intact, LPS cannot gain entrance into the bloodstream by those tight junctions. But when the cells lining the intestines (remember: the intestinal wall is only one cell thick) are damaged or become impaired and those junctions are compromised, LPS is able to pass into the systemic circulation, where it sets off an alarm and triggers inflammation. Levels of LPS in the blood are in fact indicative of both leaky gut and inflammation in general.

Researchers around the world are finally looking at LPS as playing a pivotal role in depression. After all, inflammatory markers correlate with depression, and LPS increases the production of these inflammatory chemicals. And here's where the science really shouts out to me: LPS not only compromises the gut by making it more permeable, it can also trespass the blood–brain barrier, bringing the pro-inflammatory message there as well.[18]

In 2008, the same Belgian researchers I quoted above documented a significant increase in the level of antibodies in the blood against

LPS in individuals with major depression. Interestingly, the authors commented how major depression is often accompanied by gastrointestinal symptoms. And it's one of the most logical explanations given the latest science is the fallout from a disrupted gut community. This is why we must focus on gut permeability and the tribes within the gut that are supposed to be protecting that intestinal lining.

INTESTINAL ECOLOGY

Since the outcome of the Human Genome Project in 2002, wherein scientists discovered that humans are made from a blueprint of about 23,000 genes that don't tell the whole story, we've had to begin the search for where many of our bodily processes are outsourced. If our genes are only as numerous as a worm's, then how did we get to be so unique as a species?

In just the last few years, research into the human microbiome has revolutionized medicine and our understanding of health. Essentially, all of "modern" medicine needs to go back to the drawing board. So far, it's been estimated that there are 300 trillion bacteria in our large intestine and 100 trillion on our skin.[19] The human body contains 5,000 trillion cells, with an average of 100 mitochondria per cell. The mitochondria are tiny structures within our cells (except red blood cells) that generate chemical energy in the form of ATP (adenosine triphosphate). They have their own DNA, and it's believed they originated from ancient, so-called Proteobacteria. In other words, they were once free-living unicellular organisms on Earth that ultimately found a permanent home within our cells, providing us the benefit of producing a new source of chemical energy. The mitochondria are considered a third dimension to our microbiome and have a unique relationship with the microbiome in our guts. And given their bacterial origin, there are 5,400 trillion intracellular "bacteria" outnumbering those of the gut and skin microbiomes by a factor of ten. The 2 million unique bacterial genes found in each human microbiome can make our roughly 23,000 or

so genes pale by comparison. This is where the concept of holobi-
ont comes from—that we are a living collective of microbes in and
around us, a "meta-organism" that blurs the boundaries of our own
perceived humanity.

These intestinal microbes participate in myriad different functions, from synthesizing nutrients and vitamins to helping us digest
our food and preventing us from becoming obese. The good bacteria
can also keep things in harmony by turning the spigot off of cortisol
and adrenaline—the two hormones associated with stress that can
wreak havoc on the body when they are continually flowing.[20] The
Human Microbiome Project, launched in 2008 to catalog the microorganisms living in our body, has also changed where, exactly, we
think our immune system and the fountain of mental health really
reside. Much of our immune system—in fact a great majority of it—is
located around our gut. It's called the gut-associated lymphatic tissue
(GALT), and it's significant: upward of 80 percent of our body's total
immune system is attributed to the GALT. Why is our immune system
largely stationed in the gut? Simple: the intestinal wall is the border
with the outside world, so aside from skin, it's where we have the
most chances of encountering foreign material and organisms. This
part of our immune system doesn't work in a vacuum. Much to the
contrary, it's in constant communication with every other immune
system cell throughout the body. If our immune system finds a potentially harmful substance in the gut, it will notify the rest of the
immune system to be on alert and on guard. This is also why food
choices are so fundamental to immune health, and by implication
brain health: eating the wrong thing for you could spell disaster from
the perspective of the gut-based immune system, whereas eating the
right things could literally act as a health insurance policy.[21]

The intestinal flora's jobs are extensive; the following is a summary of what the intestinal flora does for us:

▸ Create a physical barrier against potential invaders such as
harmful bacteria (pathogenic flora), sickening viruses, and inju-
rious parasites.

▶ Lend a hand in digestion and the absorption of nutrients, some of which depend on the actions of the bacteria to become assimilated into the body.

▶ Act as a detoxification machine. The gut's microbes serve as a line of defense against many toxins that reach the intestines, ultimately taking some of the load off your liver.

▶ Produce and release important enzymes and substances, including vitamins and neurotransmitters, fatty acids, and amino acids that positively affect our biology.

▶ Help us handle stress through its effects on our hormonal (endocrine) system.

▶ Dictate the immune system's activity and response. As I've mentioned, the gut *is* our biggest immune system organ. Its microbes support the immune system by controlling certain cells of the immune system and preventing autoimmunity whereby the body attacks its own tissues. They also secrete potent antibiotic substances like bacteriocins.

▶ Help regulate the body's inflammatory pathways, which in turn affect risk for virtually all manner of chronic disease.

The complexity of these relationships may be why they generally go unrecognized by doctors and the people suffering from the effects of a sick or dysfunctional microbiome. There are two keys to identifying what exactly is occurring between your gut and brain: understanding the gut's role in your immune system, and understanding the way the gut works with your hormones, specifically cortisol. When either or both of those areas are not running smoothly, the brain will be affected, and mood and memory will suffer to the point that you're labeled "depressed."

A logical question to address is how the gut and brain are linked. We've all experienced the connection through nerve-racking experiences that leave us feeling butterflies in our stomach or, worse, running to the bathroom. The vagus nerve, also known as cranial nerve X, is the longest of the twelve cranial nerves and is the primary channel of information between the 200 to 600 million nerve cells in our central nervous system and our intestinal nervous system. That's right: your nervous system comprises more than your physical brain and spinal cord. In addition to the central nervous system, you have an intestinal or enteric nervous system that is intrinsic to the gastrointestinal tract. Both the central and enteric nervous systems are created from the same tissue during fetal development, and both are connected via that vagus nerve, which extends from the brain stem to the abdomen. It forms part of the involuntary (autonomic) nervous system and directs many bodily processes that don't require conscious thinking, such as maintaining heart rate and managing digestion.

The late Dr. Nicholas Gonzalez spent three decades working at the level of the autonomic nervous system through specific nutrients, detox, and diets tailored for individual balance with clinical results in cancer and chronic disease that are unmatched the world over. He elucidated how in our body's hierarchy of systems, the master controller may very well be the nervous system implicated in traditional psychiatry, but not in the way that we have been led to believe. The autonomic nervous system exists in a state of finely calibrated balance between its two arms, the sympathetic and the parasympathetic.

The sympathetic nervous system is your body's fight-or-flight system—the one that quickens your pulse and blood pressure to shunt blood to your brain and muscles, away from digestion. It keeps you alert and mentally adept. The parasympathetic nervous system, on the other hand, is your rest and digest system that allows you to rebuild, repair, and sleep. The relationship between these two parts of the nervous system is largely determined by ancestral heritage coupled with diet and stress levels—physical, psychological, and spiritual. When we are describing depression, we are often discussing a state of parasympathetic dominance—slow, cloudy, fatigued, poor hormonal balance, and sadness. Often, however, the fight-or-flight system can be recruited under chronic stress to create a picture of "tired but wired," leaving patients to ping-pong between the parasympathetic and sympathetic states. According to the work of Weston A. Price, Francis Pottenger, William Donald Kelley, and Nicholas Gonzalez, our diets have the power to complement a nervous system that has come out of balance. In this way, the dietary recommendations in Part 2 serve to stimulate the sympathetic system to just the right degree to resolve gut, hormonal, and brain symptoms simultaneously. Bear this in mind as we discuss the multilayered effects of lifestyle changes in Part 2. For now, let's address the next question: How does your gut—and its contents—communicate inflammatory messages to the brain?

GERM FREE TO GERM FULL

The potential stress-causing effects of microbes in the gut—or the absence thereof—was first explored in the study of so-called germ-free mice. These are mice that have been specially raised without normal gut inoculation, thereby allowing scientists to study the effects of missing microbes or, conversely, exposing them to certain strains and documenting changes in behavior. A landmark study published in 2004 revealed some of the first clues to a bidirectional interaction between the brain and gut bacteria. It demonstrated that germ-free mice respond to stress in dramatic fashion, evidenced by measurable changes in brain chemistry and increased stress hormones. This condition could then be reversed by giving them a strain of the bacterium called *Bifidobacterium infantis*. Since then, there have been multiple eye-opening studies using animals to explore the relationship between the inflammation model of depression and the influence of gut bacteria.

In 2010, gastroenterologist Dr. Stephen Collins and his colleagues at McMaster University in Canada found that another strain, *Bifidobacterium longum,* could be given as a probiotic and treat anxiety-like behavior associated with chronic colitis in a mouse model of inflammatory bowel disease.[22] The mice's behavioral changes were so severe that Collins and his team went on to perform an investigation of the ability of intestinal bacteria to influence the brain and behavior. Additional animal experiments in Collins's lab further confirmed the researchers' initial observations. By manipulating the intestinal microbiota of mice, he demonstrated that gut bacteria can influence anxiety-like behaviors. Some of the most remarkable discoveries have come from fecal transplants, procedures in which researchers swap the intestinal microbiota from one mouse to another using strained stool samples that contain a particular bacterial profile that can be transplanted into another mouse's gut much in the way you'd transplant a heart. In the swap, researchers noted a change in behavior. Put another way, a once anxious mouse adopted the less anxious behavior of the donor mouse and vice versa. A growing amount of preclinical evidence from other laboratories continues to underscore the relationship between the gut microbiota, stress, and anxiety-related behaviors.[23] And now the race is on to understand how these connections work in humans.

Dr. Emeran Mayer is a gastroenterologist at UCLA where he is also a professor of medicine and directs the Center for Neurobiology of Stress. He has devoted much of his recent research to understanding the communication between the gut and brain. He points out that while studying germ-free mice can help answer specific black-and-white questions such as whether the gut microbes are involved in the stress response, there are limitations to the clinical relevance of these studies. After all, these animals show abnormalities in brain, immune, and gastrointestinal function. "The magnitude of these effects may be developmentally dictated, as studies suggest there are specific critical windows in which microbiota play a key role in sculpting behavior," states a 2015 article in the *Journal of the American Medical Association*.[24]

This is a key point. As Dr. Collins also noted in the same *JAMA* article, "Anything that interferes with the microbial colonization process early on can set the scene for trouble down the road, and the declining robustness of the microbiome as one ages is likely to be a major determinant of healthy aging."[25] Such a bold statement gives credence to the finding that maternal stress, infections, and the use of antibiotics can ravage the microbiome during important but vulnerable prenatal and neonatal periods when the gut is first colonized by the mother's microbiome. These disruptions ultimately affect normal neurodevelopment and may even increase the risk of neuropsychiatric disorders including depression later in life.[26]

My patients are often surprised when I ask them where they were born and whether or not hospital walls and their mother's vaginal canal were key players in their emergence. But how we are born sets the ultimate stage for the microbiome. It actually starts in utero through the transfer of our mother's gut bacteria, and then more microbes are added to the mix when we descend through the vaginal canal and are breast-fed. This is nature's way of preparing a baby for the mother's world. Children who miss out on this microbial baptism because they are born via C-section, receive antibiotics during the birth process (intrapartum), and go home dominated by the skin flora of other adults have been shown in many high-profile studies to live with an increased risk for allergies, eczema, asthma, and some forms of cancer. Even those born vaginally in the hospital are more likely to suffer allergies because of colonization by hospital flora such as *Clostridium difficile.*

In 2013, the *Canadian Medical Association Journal* stated the facts squarely when a group of researchers referred to the gut microbiota as being a "super organ" with "diverse roles in health and disease."[27] In a related commentary about the study, Dr. Rob Knight, a world leader in the study of the microbiome who is a professor at UC San Diego School of Medicine, said: "Children born by cesarean delivery or fed with formula may be at increased risk of a variety of conditions later in life; both processes alter the gut microbiota in healthy infants, which could be the mechanism for the increased risk."[28]

For the record, C-sections are medically necessary under certain rare circumstances, and the trend lately has been to minimize the risks of this intervention, both acute risks to the mother and long-term risks to the baby. Dr. Martin Blaser, who directs New York University's Human Microbiome Program and is the author of *Missing Microbes,* notes that a third of infants born in the United

States today are born by C-section, which reflects a 50 percent increase since 1996.[29] Every woman who gives birth by C-section also receives antibiotics, which means all babies born this way start life with a huge insult to their developing microbiome.[30] Later in the book I'll provide explicit details on preventing and overcoming a C-section and speak to both expecting mothers and those who've already given birth. And as you can likely guess, I'm a huge advocate for breast-feeding and will discuss what you can do to support a healthy supply.

PALEO-DEFICIT DISORDER[31]

Diminishing the foundational importance of conception, pregnancy, and birth is just one of the ways that we have shaped our adult health for the worse. We've wandered so far off the path, one might worry that it's too late to learn what a healthy gut actually looks like. Contrary to what you might think, the dividing line between "good" and "bad" bacteria—tribes that benefit you and others that can maim—isn't that clear yet. It's more about the overall diversity and the ratios of strains relative to one another. In the right quantity, certain strains that probably have positive effects on health can turn into villains. The notorious bacteria *Escherichia coli,* for instance, produces vitamin K but can also cause severe illness.

In 2014, a collaboration of researchers from around the world published findings in *Nature* that compared gut microbiota from a community of human hunter-gatherers, the Hadza of Tanzania, with Italian urban controls.[32] The Hadza showed much higher levels of microbial richness and biodiversity and marked gender differences based on dietary nuances between men and women. And it turns out that as more samples of hunter-gatherer microbiomes come into the science lab—profiles of the microbes found in the intestines of traditional societies like those of the Yanomami of Venezuela and the Matsés of Peru—the more we must acknowledge there isn't one single, universal microbiome that's "healthy."

To the dismay of people who like to label certain strains of bacteria as "good" and "bad," the Hadza guts, for example, contain almost no *Bifidobacteria,* a microbial group that is generally viewed as healthy by Western science and comprises up to 10 percent of a Western gut microbiome. The Hadza, Yanomami, and Matsés also harbor a lot more *spirochetes,* a fiber-loving group of bacteria that includes the species responsible for syphilis and yaws (a bacterial infection common in tropical regions). These differences clearly aren't unhealthy, as these people enjoy levels of freedom from chronic disease we can only fantasize about. Their microbiota reflect the conditions in that particular corner of the world, its food supplies, water, climate, and more. The bottom line is that we don't necessarily know what is optimal, so we can only support optimal diet to adjust our internal ecology. Diets dictate microbiota over other exposures (including copious pill popping of probiotics), which is why modern hunter-gatherers even from different continents have similar microbiomes.

Dr. William Parker of Duke University has spent time researching another fascinating angle to the microbiome: the modern-day absence of helminths, eukaryotic organisms such as whipworms and tapeworms, which offered positive effects on our immunity over our shared evolution, but have been long since wiped out of our gutscape by industrialization.[33]

We know that we have coevolved with the microbial world over millions of years, and that this partnered dance is contextualized by native cultural practices, nutritional traditions, and the greater network of the flora and fauna in the immediate surroundings. As urban dwellers, however, we suffer from "Paleo deficit disorder," a term coined by Alan C. Logan and his colleagues in their fascinating two-part treatise on how we have strayed from the stimulus our genes expect. They write:

> We wonder could this collective deficit manifest in a "disorder," a sort of paleo-deficit disorder, that while not pathological per se, taps into unrealized quality of life,

empathy, perspective taking, low-grade anxiety, psychological distress, resiliency, and negative mental outlook? Could this deficit accelerate an individual toward the checkmarks required for medicalized diagnoses? Might the collective deficit in "Paleolithic experiences" compromise an individual's ability to maintain optimal emotional health and by extension, prevent optimal health of neighborhoods, cities, societies, and nations, especially those undergoing rapid urbanization?[34]

As I have mentioned, we are learning that we are not plants that can be sustained with fluorescent light, recirculated air, and soil fertilizer. Our vitality is inextricably connected to and dependent on our greater ecosystem. This ecosystem includes our food and its ecosystems, but extends to movement in green space, early daytime exposure to light, contact with the earth, and communities—all strategies you'll learn more about in Part 2. Logan explores microbiologist René Dubos's tenets:

> . . . modern disconnects from ancestral influences—natural environments, traditional dietary practices, and incidental exposure to non-pathogenic microbes—would make itself known in health and well-being statistics (or outcomes related to humanness such as empathy) . . . Dubos argued that because humans are very adaptable, the relationship between an evolutionary mismatch and erosion of health would be stealth-like; there would be only minimal awareness of the association, especially early on in the era of high technology and urbanization.[35]

Let's raise that awareness, and do what we can to resolve our Paleo deficits. Otherwise, we will only continue to suffer from an evolutionary mismatch that fuels debilitating mood disorders, not to mention all manner of chronic illnesses rooted in inflammation run amok.

TOP GUT BOMBS IN OUR MODERN
LIFESTYLES THAT DRIVE INFLAMMATION

I get asked all the time about which daily encounters can adversely affect the microbiome and how we can rebalance our gut ecology. Both questions can be answered through one word: diet. It's a major determinant of what bugs are most active in our guts, and how those bugs respond to agents that can cause inflammation.

Plenty of studies have begun to look at how our diet may be chiefly responsible for both increased gut permeability and loss of bacterial diversity—both of which bridge the gap between diet and risk for depression.[36] What the science is revealing is that people who adhere to a protocol that's rich in healthy, anti-inflammatory fats and proteins enjoy significantly lower rates of depression. Conversely, a diet high in carbs and sugar is fanning the flames of inflammation. We can even examine the effects of ingredients like gluten and fructose on the body's inflammatory pathways, the latter of which has been shown to increase LPS in the bloodstream by 40 percent.[37] But this can be reversed back to normal when the balance of gut microbes is shifted, proving that the elevated LPS from the fructose is related to changes in the gut bacteria. Fructose is naturally found in fruit, but most of the fructose we consume is from manufactured sources. Our caveman ancestors did eat fructose in the context of whole fruit, but only during certain times of the year when it was available; we haven't yet evolved to handle the prodigious amounts of industry isolated fructose we consume today. High-fructose corn syrup now represents 42 percent of all caloric sweeteners. And this firmly connects our Western diet, so high in processed fructose, to soaring rates of depression. It also helps explain the connection between obesity and depression.

Although restoring optimal gut flora requires a variety of interventions, it begins simply with a grain- and dairy-free diet that eliminates sugar and genetically modified (GM) foods invariably contaminated with Roundup herbicide (glyphosate). When you follow my protocol in Part 2, you'll be making those adjustments to your diet and learning about other dietary and lifestyle strategies that can help optimize healthy intestinal tribes. My patients know I'm a bit of a food fanatic and that I won't see them for a second consult until they've followed my food protocol (the same one in this book), with no exceptions. Dietary change is step one, because we can change the microbiota dominance within seventy-two hours of simple changes to eliminate potential triggers to the immune system and rebalance the gut flora.

Below is a summary of the top gut bombs. We'll be further exploring these ingredients and others commonly found in our kitchens and bathroom cabinets in upcoming chapters, but I wanted to give you a little primer here to start you thinking about the biggest everyday villains.

Gluten

Gluten, from the Latin word *glue,* is a protein found in wheat, but you can also find gluten-like proteins, known as prolamins, in barley (hordein), rye (secalin), and corn (zein). These are among the most inflammatory ingredients of the modern era. While a small percentage of the population is highly sensitive to gluten and suffers from celiac disease, it's possible for anyone to have a negative albeit undetected reaction. Gluten in wheat is made up of two main groups of proteins, the glutenins and the gliadins. You can be sensitive to either of these proteins or to one of the twelve different smaller units that make up gliadin. A reaction to any of these could lead to inflammation with both biological and psychological consequences.

Often processed with engineered oils in refined foods, gluten can be a brain and body poison. Its havoc begins in the gut, where it promotes intestinal permeability by upregulating a compound called zonulin. Gluten's "sticky" attribute interferes with the breakdown and absorption of nutrients, which leads to poorly digested food that can then sound the alarm on the immune system, which results in an assault on the lining of the small intestine and more inflammation. Those who experience symptoms of gluten sensitivity complain of abdominal pain, nausea, diarrhea, constipation, and intestinal distress. Many people who don't experience these blatant signs of gastrointestinal trouble could nevertheless be experiencing a silent attack. According to notable gluten researcher Dr. Marios Hadjivassiliou, "gluten sensitivity can be primarily, and at times, exclusively, a neurological disease."[38]

The neurologic effects of gluten intolerance include depression, seizures, headaches, multiple sclerosis/demyelination, anxiety, symptoms associated with ADHD diagnoses, ataxia (loss of control of bodily movements), and nerve damage.[39] In fact, the research site GreenMedInfo.com has cataloged more than two hundred conditions linked to gluten-containing wheat consumption, and of the twenty-two modes of toxicity, neurotoxicity was found top on the list. When I recommend a gluten-free diet to patients, they sometimes tell me they have already been tested for celiac disease, the autoimmune disorder famously associated with gluten sensitivity, and they don't have it. Know that there are limitations in the conventional testing currently available. Most physicians order a celiac panel that only tests for a small number of the potential immune responses to this food. But gluten consists of six sets of chromosomes capable of producing greater than 23,000 proteins. So this testing may be too limited to the point of being useless. In one study, an inflammatory gut response was noted in the intestinal cells of healthy volunteers, suggesting that gluten may cause reactions in *everyone*.[40]

Dairy

I used to be a dairy addict. When my naturopath asked me to give up gluten and dairy six years ago, it was about two more years before I stopped fantasizing about cheese, milk, ice cream, ricotta (yes, I'm Italian), and yogurt. It turns out we have a decent explanation for the deep pleasure associated with dairy and its best friend, wheat. It's the morphine-like exorphin compounds found in these foods, which interact with opiate receptors in the brain and other bodily tissues.

There is a burgeoning literature in psychiatry that supports immune responses to the protein casein in dairy, primarily cow, as playing a role in conditions ranging from depression to schizophrenia.

This is not to say that dairy is a problem for everyone, or that all dairy is a problem for some. In my experience, reintroduction of dairy after a month of elimination is enough to tell you which camp you fall in. In fact, I have had patients report vomiting upon reexposure—to something they had eaten daily for decades! So to start I'll be asking you to quit dairy for at least thirty days and show you how to return to it if you are able (and which type of dairy is OK; there's a difference!).

GMOs

In the past few years, many scientists have begun to explore the impact of herbicides such as Monsanto's Roundup (glyphosate) on the human gut microbiome. Glyphosate is used in more than 750 products and plays a large role in the production of genetically modified crops such as soy, canola, and corn. Unfortunately, it is even found in non-GMO foods like wheat and oats because it is used as a pre-harvest desiccant (a drying agent to prime the soil for a new crop). As it turns out, this chemical is very active in disrupting beneficial bacteria via its impact on the shikimate pathway, which is an important metabolic route that many microorganisms and plants use to manufacture certain amino acids—amino acids we need but that we cannot produce ourselves because our biology doesn't include this pathway.[41] By imbalancing this flora, pesticides and herbicides disrupt the production of essential amino acids such as tryptophan, a serotonin precursor, and promote production of *p*-Cresol, a compound that interferes with metabolism of other xenobiotics, or environmental chemicals, making the individual more vulnerable to their toxic effects. Even vitamin D_3 activation in the liver may be affected negatively by glyphosate's effect on liver enzymes, potentially explaining epidemic levels of vitamin D deficiency.

The scientific literature also contains evidence that insecticidal toxins, such as Bt-toxin, which is prominent in genetically altered corn, is transferred into the blood of pregnant women and their fetuses, and that glyphosate herbicide transfers to breast milk. Genetic modification of foods, in addition to guaranteeing exposure to pesticides and herbicides, entails risks of gene transfer to human gut bacteria, turning them into pesticide-producing factories.

Artificial Sugars

In the next chapter, I'll go into detail about the impact sugar can have on your entire physiology and mental wellness. Here I want to highlight the effects of sugar's evil twins: the Equals and Splendas of the world. Indeed, the fact that our gut bacteria are affected by the sugar we consume has just recently been revealed from studies done on *artificial* sweeteners. The human body cannot digest artificial sweeteners, which is why they have no calories. But they still must pass through our gastrointestinal tract. For a long time we assumed that artificial sweeteners were, for the most part, inert ingredients in their effect on our physiology. Far from it. In 2014, a bombshell paper published in *Nature* proved that artificial sugars affect healthy gut bacteria in ways that lead to metabolic syndromes in the human host, such as insulin resistance and diabetes, contributing to the same overweight and obesity epidemic they were marketed to provide a solution for.[42]

Antibiotics

Most women who have developed a yeast infection after taking a round of antibiotics are familiar with the idea that antibiotics kill important regulatory bacteria. They think "I'll just eat a little extra yogurt or maybe take a probiotic" (to restore dramatic changes that are not easily undone). Antibiotics, invented and studied before our knowledge of the microbiome and the role of mitochondrial dysfunction in chronic disease, have never been adequately studied for safety. We are learning that the effects of exposure to antibiotics on gut bacteria can persist for months after treatment and sometimes result in permanent disability. In fact, HormonesMatter.com has extensively documented neurological and psychiatric conditions following common antibiotics like fluoroquinolones (such as Cipro).

Antibiotics are a prime example of how our antiquated concepts are driving the recklessness of conventional medicine. They are employed in a framework of us against them rather than the emerging reality that we need microbes and must work *with* them for optimal health. In this way, antibiotics, like vaccines, are like drinking poison to kill the enemy.

With 40 percent of adults and 70 percent of children (and billions of industrially farmed animals) taking antibiotics, I ask my patients to opt out of this statistical nightmare. I ask them to support their immunity naturally through lifestyle medicine, to shed their fear of infection that has little chance of killing a healthy individual, and to support their system through a nutrient-dense diet rich in vitamins A, D, C, and the use of natural antimicrobials and immune modulators. Protect your bugs and they'll protect you. I'll show you how to do that in Part 2.

NSAIDs and Proton-Pump Inhibitors (Acid-Reflux Drugs)

You may think of ibuprofen as an innocuous over-the-counter comfort for easing aches and pains. The same goes for modern-day antacids such as Nexium and Prevacid. Some people are so lulled into a sense of safety and efficacy that they keep these pills in their purses and nightstands for everyday use. But as we'll see in Chapter 5, these drugs are far from harmless, especially when it comes to our intestinal tract and its microbial inhabitants. Briefly, they can promote bleeding, deplete nutrients, increase intestinal permeability, aggravate the immune system, and trigger autoimmune and inflammatory processes. Need I say more? I will: They can also sustain dysbiosis, an imbalance in the microbiome—the delicate microbiome that's required to prevent such insults to the lining and the immune system!

IT'S ALL CONNECTED

I can't reiterate this enough: the interconnectedness of the gut, brain, and immune and hormonal systems is exceedingly difficult to unravel. Until we begin to recognize this complex relationship, we will not be able to prevent or effectively intervene in depression. For true healing and prevention, we must work every day to send our bodies the message that we are not being attacked, we are not in danger, and we are well-nourished, well-supported, and calm.

As a society, we can begin to think about protecting the microbiome by demedicalizing birth and infant nutrition; as individuals, we can avoid antibiotics, NSAIDs, gluten-containing grains, processed synthetic hormone-laden dairy, genetically modified foods, and nonorganic foods. Promising interventions for depression from a gut-brain perspective include probiotics, fermented foods, natural fats and eliciting the relaxation response for optimal digestion, anti-inflammatory, and insulin sensitizing effects. This is termed a psychoneuroimmunological approach, and it is likely to represent the future of mental health care. This approach will compel clinicians and researchers alike to recognize both the inexorable interplay of various bodily systems and our connectedness to the environmental ecosystem in and around us.

CHAPTER 4

The Great Psychiatric Pretenders

*Two Common, Resolvable Conditions That Can
Lead to a Psychiatric Diagnosis*

Are your "healthy eating" habits stealing your vibrancy?

Is your "normal" thyroid test hiding a secret source of depression?

Sometimes it takes a personal health crisis to force a conventional doctor to stop, look, and listen to another voice. That's exactly what happened to me. I was a traditionally trained physician who bumped up against the severe limitations of orthodox medicine and was compelled to cross over to the other side and eventually leave everything I had learned about treatment behind. It was a mixed blessing. You see, I was that girl who could eat whatever I wanted, shun exercise, stay up late, and never gain weight. And I did that for the better part of thirty years. All throughout my medical residency, I ate at McDonald's and White Castle, drank Red Bulls, and kept Snickers bars in my purse to sustain me on little sleep. Before trying to start a family, I took birth control pills, ibuprofen for the occasional headache, and even beta blockers for my inexplicably racing heart. I welcomed my first daughter during my fellowship and was back at work within three weeks, with lots of energy to boot. My pregnancy weight melted off quickly and I felt pretty good despite my eighty-hour workweek.

Nine months later, though, I was in a totally different state. I felt like I was losing my mind. I loved being a mom and juggling the new balancing act of my home life and working at both the hospital and my budding private practice, but I was so fatigued that my limbs felt as if they were made of lead. And I was experiencing disturbing lapses in my mental abilities, becoming absentminded in a way that was completely new to me: repeatedly locking myself out of my office, forgetting my long-standing ATM PIN, double-booking patients, and mailing checks to cabdrivers on days when I'd left my wallet behind (compassionate souls). This behavior was not good for my career or my confidence as a new mother. Even though I wasn't feeling down, as a psychiatrist and postpartum patient, I knew that many of these symptoms could be categorized under the blanket diagnosis of depression, which called for the reflexive panacea: the antidepressant.

Lab tests from a routine physical finally identified the problem: my thyroid, a vitally important master gland that produces hormones to influence almost all of the metabolic processes in the body, including those that relate to mood and memory, had come under attack. My testing showed signs of what's called Hashimoto's thyroiditis, an autoimmune disorder that causes the body to target its own thyroid tissue for destruction. In this disease the thyroid swells with inflammation, tissue is destroyed, and the gland underperforms. (In fact, Hashimoto's was the first autoimmune disease to be recognized, initially described in 1912.)[1] My doctor explained that it was a chronic disease, gave me not one word of advice on how I might have come to this point or how to ameliorate the condition without drugs, and wrote me a prescription for a synthetic thyroid hormone I would have to take for the rest of my life. No big deal.

But it was a big deal for me. I'd never been sick in my life, and now I was confronted with my first diagnosis and the prospect of lifelong treatment. I knew from my perinatal research that thyroid autoimmunity (even with normal hormone levels) can lead to miscarriage and preterm birth, and I knew that I wanted to expand my family. I'm generally rather suspicious of other people's recommendations, doctors included, and I've always been a bit of a rebel. So I went to a wonderful naturopath who ushered me into the gentle, hopeful world of self-repair. I plunged into my own investigative work, not only as a physician myself but as a newly desperate patient. And I soon discovered that at the heart of my struggle, it wasn't fundamentally a thyroid problem at all—it was a serious glitch in my immune system triggered by postpartum shifts, chronic gut imbalance, and suboptimal dietary patterns (*ahem*: those Big Macs and energy drinks were starting to exact their revenge). It was all manifesting in thyroid dysfunction. There probably were underlying blood sugar issues as well, for all that processed junk food had to be killing me softly. Suffice it to say the experience made me appreciate the interconnectedness of all systems in the body. The silver lining was that it became an experience that ultimately made it possible to help many other women who are in the same position today, and to serve as a gatekeeper, keeping them from the psychiatric pill mill.

Seven years and another healthy pregnancy later, I now know that thyroid dysregulation stemming from an immune system response is a common but often unidentified cause of depression and anxiety (and you don't have to be a new mother to experience thyroid problems). I also know that there are clear, evidence-based strategies for restoring thyroid function, *no prescription needed*. I found a way to lift myself out of the forgetful fog. No sooner did I tweak my diet, commence a specific dietary supplement regimen, and start exercising regularly and meditating than I achieved total relief (resolution of antibody levels and healthy thyroid levels). It's the program that this book's protocol is based on.

Don't get me wrong: my personal journey hasn't always been easy, and it took almost two years of merciless discipline to completely resolve my problems. I've had to learn more about human biology than I could have ever anticipated needing (especially as a traditionally trained psychiatrist), and this new knowledge completely upended almost everything I'd studied during my long medical training spanning more than a decade. I was forced to *unlearn* most of what had cost me hundreds of thousands of dollars, sleepless nights, undue stress, and indentured servitude. Putting the information into practice has been a true labor of self-love. But I've reaped my reward, not just in mental stability but also in excellent physical health. And I want nothing more than for you to be able to do the same for yourself.

By this point in the book, you know that depression is far from simply a brain disorder. But did you know that some very ordinary conditions that go undiagnosed can actually seem like textbook psychiatric disorders? They are what I call the psychiatric pretenders, and a misbehaving thyroid—not misbehaving brain chemicals—is among the most common one in women today. In fact, an underperforming thyroid (hypothyroidism) is one of the most underdiagnosed conditions in America, yet it's incredibly common, especially in women. Upward of 20 percent of all women have a "lazy" thyroid, but only half of those women get diagnosed (and this diagnosis isn't as easy as you'd think). The other pretender—blood sugar imbalance—is also endemic today, and few doctors make the connection between being on the verge of diabetes (if not already diabetic) and depression. But as you'll soon learn, these two pretenders share a lot in common.

MAYHEM IN THE THYROID

Melissa was just thirty-one years old with no previous psychiatric history when she came to me complaining of agitation, a racing heart, insomnia, and anxiety. Another psychiatrist had given her prescriptions for the antianxiety drug Ativan and the antidepressant Zoloft. But she was hoping to avoid taking these medications and looked to me for better solutions. The first thing I did was order tests to pinpoint any abnormalities in her physiology. Although her thyroid stimulating hormone (TSH) levels were normal using the routine test most doctors order, I found out she had grossly elevated thyroid autoantibodies from routine tests most doctors *don't* order.

This meant that her body's immune system was attacking its own thyroid tissue. It was the first stage of Hashimoto's thyroiditis, a diagnosis that can predate a formal diagnosis by up to seven years.

As I mentioned, hypothyroidism, a condition in which your thyroid gland doesn't produce enough of certain key thyroid hormones, is epidemic among women today. Nearly 60 million Americans, mostly women, have some type of thyroid problem and are prescribed synthetic thyroid hormones such as Synthroid. Most of us never think about our thyroid, but this butterfly-shaped gland located at the base of the neck has important functions, including the production of hormones that regulate metabolism (including the creation of new mitochondria, our cells' energy packers), controlling protein synthesis, and adjusting the body's sensitivity to other hormones. The thyroid is also involved in detoxification, growth functions, immunity, and cognition.

Many chemicals and food additives can interfere with thyroid function, from commercial soda (which contains chemicals called emulsifiers) and plastics (which contain the synthetic chemical bisphenol A and its relatives) to tap water (which often contains fluoride) and mercury from large fish swimming in our contaminated seas. Specifically, the thyroid is responsible for producing what's called T0, T1, T2, T3, and T4. The first three (T0, T1, and T2) are hormone precursors and by-products of making thyroid hormone; as such, they don't actually act on the thyroid hormone receptor and play a role we have yet to fully elucidate. The two most active thyroid hormones are T3 and T4. Most of the T4, the storage form of thyroid hormone, is converted into its active form, T3, in tissues around the body including the brain. This is a process dependent on specialized enzymes, optimal cortisol (your stress hormone), and certain nutrients such as iron, iodine, zinc, magnesium, selenium, B vitamins, vitamin C, and vitamin D.

Given that the thyroid hormones are essentially the metabolic lifeline for every cell in the body, it makes sense to take care of such a critical source of health. But thyroid health is often just an afterthought at best. When the thyroid's active hormone is deficient or poorly functioning, we can experience an array of depression-like symptoms, including fatigue, constipation, hair loss, low mood, foggy thinking, feeling cold all the time, low metabolism, weight gain, dry skin, muscle aches, and an intolerance for exercise. You're wearing socks to bed, pooping only once a week, and penciling in your eyebrows because the hair has gone missing. Postpartum thyroiditis, what I experienced, is typically preceded by a period of functional *hyper*thyroidism, whereby you can feel overenergized and suffer from insomnia, diarrhea, anxiety, and precipitous weight loss. These are the women who "bounce back" quickly after the baby, only to be peeling themselves off the ground nine months later. Hyperthyroidism, when the gland produces too much thyroid hormone, is rarer, but also has negative effects on the body including the triggering of heart and bone problems.

Are You Really a Mental Patient?

So how much of what we call mental illness is actually driven by the thyroid and, one step back, the immune system? In my experience, a vast majority is. Scientists have long known about the relationship between a dysfunctional thyroid and symptoms of depression. Among the first papers to come out showing the connection between "symptomless" autoimmune thyroiditis and depression was one published in 1982 by Dr. Mark S. Gold and his colleagues.[2] Gold is a world-renowned addiction expert who has had a long career studying and researching the effects of drugs on brain and behavior; he has also done work on how undetected dysfunctions in the body can manifest in depressive symptoms. Ten years after Gold's landmark paper, the *British Medical Journal* published a paper that further established the relationship between thyroid dysfunction and depression. And this relationship continues to be validated: in 2015, the peer-reviewed journal *European Archives of Psychiatry and Clinical Neuroscience* published an original paper that further confirmed the association between autoimmune thyroiditis and depression. The authors wrote: "Our study demonstrates a strong association between [thyroid autoantibody] levels, which are considered to be of diagnostic value for autoimmune thyroiditis . . . with uni- or bipolar depression."[3]

But doctors today often don't consider the thyroid when a woman comes in with these vague but insidious complaints.[4] Rather than order tests to nail the real problem, they instead write a prescription. Unfortunately, finding a problem in the thyroid is something you often have to go digging for.

Even when doctors do test the thyroid, they don't always get accurate results. This is because standard tests look at only one hormone in the blood that is produced by the brain's pituitary gland: TSH. Normally the pituitary gland releases TSH in response to a low thyroid hormone level, so an elevated TSH level would typically suggest an underactive thyroid. But for many women, this is akin to keeping the lights off in a dark room and saying you can't find your lost keys.

The problem with the established reference ranges for what's considered normal and abnormal is that the cutoffs on thyroid function tests are based on an unscreened population sample likely inclusive of those with undiagnosed thyroid dysfunction. Put simply, the reference ranges are misleading, so there's a lot of underdiagnosis— many people whose tests come back normal in fact have a damaged thyroid. Labeling a certain reference range as normal implies a degree of accuracy the tests cannot support. We all have our own individual, slightly different set point for what's considered normal or abnormal for thyroid functionality, something the tests cannot factor into the equation.

Doctors don't know how to scrutinize the whole picture. They rarely look at free hormone levels—levels of thyroid hormones in the blood that aren't bound to proteins and that are typically missed with routine testing. They don't appreciate the relevance of the immune system as a lever for disease reversal. So they don't screen for thyroid antibodies and they don't change their "gold-standard" treatment, which is a one-size-fits-all synthetic thyroid hormone. No wonder Synthroid is the most prescribed drug today.[5] But it's rarely the solution. My protocol can help return thyroid function to normal, and alternatives for those who truly need supplemental thyroid hormone do exist. (See Chapter 10, where I also cover exactly which tests to ask for in identifying an underperforming thyroid that go beyond the standard thyroid test.)

Conventional medicine fails to appreciate the interplay between many easy-to-compartmentalize factors. And when a patient isn't properly diagnosed or doesn't respond to a prescription for thyroid hormone, well then . . . she must need a psychiatrist. After all, her symptoms—brain fog, fatigue, insomnia, agitation, anxiety— correlate with depression and her TSH levels are "normal." Treating these women with antidepressants is like putting a bandage over a splinter that's gotten buried in the skin. It's missing an opportunity to resolve it at the root. And it's a telling example of how traditional medicine can make grave mistakes.

How does the thyroid affect mental health? First, it helps to understand that thyroid health is so much more than pumping out a hormonal product—it involves a sophisticated conversation between the brain, thyroid gland, hormones, and the receiving cells and tissues. In fact, we can't even address thyroid health without looking at the mitochondria, the tiny organelles in your cells that contain their own DNA and are responsible for a laundry list of chores ranging from creating life-sustaining energy to determining the time of a cell's death. As such, mitochondria have increasingly become the focus of chronic disease research, and the keeper of your mitochondria is your thyroid hormone. This is why when your thyroid isn't performing optimally you can experience the array of symptoms I listed above. What's more, the thyroid's functionality is at the mercy of the stress hormone cortisol, which is produced by your adrenal glands and signaled by your brain.

For me, the question to ask is why adrenal output is abnormal. Why is the brain shutting down cortisol secretion, leaving patients tired but wired? When we are trying to resurrect thyroid function, we simply can't ignore the adrenals. Adrenals are little glands that sit over our kidneys and make a variety of hormones and neurochemicals that help us respond to everyday demands. These substances that govern much of our biological stress-response system include cortisol, DHEA, aldosterone, norepinephrine, and epinephrine. For optimal thyroid hormone conversion and effect, the pattern of cortisol over the course of the day must be optimized. For this reason I have my patients test their cortisol levels throughout the day (see page 221); testing cortisol is necessary for seeing the bigger picture of thyroid function. Ideal cortisol patterns go beyond stress management. As I'll cover in Part 2, a low-sugar diet and the addition of certain anti-inflammatory vitamins and herbs are additional vital tools in taking back full control of your health.

When we consider which stressors recruit the adrenals, we must consider the following offenders:

Birth control pills

The synthetic hormones in these popular pills effectively lower available thyroid hormone in the body (even though your thyroid tests comes back as normal) by elevating thyroid-binding globulin. In plain speak, thyroid-binding globulin is a protein that binds to thyroid hormone in the bloodstream. When thyroid-binding globin goes up, your thyroid levels go down. Birth control pills have also been demonstrated to promote inflammation while depleting critical nutrients and antioxidants. I'll cover more about birth control pills in the next chapter. I want my patients off birth control pills, and I suggest other options such as condoms, non-hormonal IUDs, and the rhythm method.

Gluten

As I described in the previous chapter, the "sticky" proteins found in wheat, as well as gluten-like prolamin proteins in barley, rye, and corn, have both direct effects on the brain and indirect effects on the rest of the body. The thyroid gland in particular takes a hit. It's well documented that sensitivity to gluten-containing grains, which can oftentimes go unnoticed and undiagnosed, drives both celiac disease and Hashimoto's thyroiditis, among more than two hundred validated health conditions. Part of the reason for this link is the fact that the thyroid itself contains amino acid sequences (i.e., proteins) that resemble those found in gluten, which is why the immune system can become confused and start pouncing on the thyroid as if it were a foreign invader. In 2001, *The American Journal of Gastroenterology* published a remarkable study showing that individuals with the worst reactions to gluten—people with celiac disease—have three times the risk of thyroid dysfunction, and eliminating gluten can totally resolve the symptoms.[6] And studies dating back to the 1980s show a strong association between untreated celiac disease and depression.

Fluoride

Historically, fluoride was used to suppress thyroid function in patients with an overactive thyroid. It interferes with multiple aspects of the thyroid's tissues, disrupts normal hormone physiology, and both displaces iodine and depletes selenium, two critically essential elements for thyroid function. Fluoride is ubiquitous today, found in our drinking water, medications, nonstick cookware, and toothpaste. Recent research shows that fluoride in water not only increases risk of thyroid illness by 30 percent, but it may not prevent cavities—the main reason it's added to water in the first place.[7] I'll help you minimize your exposure when I outline my protocol.

Endocrine disruptors

Since you were in your mother's womb you've been exposed to thousands of environmental chemicals, many of which can disturb normal physiology. Today's industrial and agricultural chemicals such as phthalates, flame retardants, and PCBs are pervasive toxicants that interfere with the thyroid's biology. These toxicants, which we'll be exploring in Chapter 5, also derail hormone balance in general, promote inflammation, and negatively stimulate the immune system.

The thyroid is a canary in the coal mine. In our fast-paced, nutrient-depleted world that's filled with toxic substances, your thyroid gland may be the first to come under siege. And while you may not feel the attack in your thyroid per se, you'll definitely feel it in your mood. Supporting a healthy thyroid is truly an exercise in holistic medicine. And it starts with supporting the immune system so it doesn't go rogue on the body's own tissues and manifest as symptoms of depression. And another huge reason to correct autoimmune thyroid dysfunction is to lessen the risk of developing other autoimmune disorders such as arthritis, lupus, and multiple sclerosis.

With these exposures, the challenge is knowing if you are at risk of experiencing adverse effects and how much exposure will trigger your body to respond negatively. We live in an overstimulated world, and it is difficult to predict whose systems are going to rebel against it. Connecting the dots between your immune system and mental health may seem convoluted and difficult at first, but not after you come to appreciate the direct, intimate relationship shared between these two networks in the body. Let's go there now.

It's the Immune System, Dummy

As with any living thing on this beautiful and strange planet, our body has a will to survive as an individual organism, alongside billions of other organisms that compete for some of the same resources. In addition to the classic flight-or-fight response that we are all born with to help survive our encounters with predators in the outside world, the human body has also developed methods to attack and kill whatever threatens our survival from the inside. Our immune systems' cells are constantly surveying the environment to detect organisms and molecules that are foreign and potentially hostile, and it does so by recognizing surface structures that identify them as "other."[8]

As babies, our immune systems are deliberately clamped down so that we can learn, from breast milk, what to respond to, but just as important what *not* to respond to. Levels of stress hormone in pregnancy and even during the lactation period repeatedly convey important information to a baby about the nature of its new home.[9] It is this complex partnership with the microbial world that a mother must teach her infant, and has for millions of years.

Remember: gut-associated lymphatic tissue, or GALT, is responsible for upward of 80 percent of our body's first line of defense. The idea that the gut-based immune system and your mental health work in tandem is not something your doctor is likely thinking about, so he won't ask what you're eating or inquire about your digestion when you come in complaining of classic symptoms of depression. But if something is askew in your immune system, it can most definitely trigger psychiatric symptoms because of the intricate relationships shared by the immune system, gut, hormonal glands, and brain. Many popular Western foods contain ingredients that cause far-reaching though mostly unrecognized immune system effects, sometimes entirely *outside* of the gut (so those perfect poops don't mean you don't have gut issues). Seemingly minor immune responses in the gut come with downstream mood and memory effects, but again you might not necessarily feel those initial reactions. I'll cover the top ingredients that trigger immune responses in Chapter 7 (for a sneak peek, see the sidebar on page 107). These are foods we humans were not designed to eat, and *no one should be consuming them*. I will go so far as to call them downright toxic to the body. The good news is that it's a relatively simple matter to eliminate these potential immune triggers from your diet. Some people will also have intolerances or allergies to other foods that they will have to avoid in their diet, even though I recommend them on this program. Nightshade vegetables, eggs, and tree nuts, for example, are problematic for a small number of people for which substitutions should be made. If you have these types of food allergies, chances are you already know it and will be able to modify the dietary protocol appropriately.

TOP (TOXIC) INGREDIENTS TO ELIMINATE RIGHT AWAY

▶ Gluten-containing proteins (found in wheat, barley, and rye)

▶ Most forms of sugar (refined sugar, high-fructose corn syrup, and artificial sugars, including the Equals and Splendas of the world)

▶ Nonorganic and genetically modified (GM) foods such as corn, soy, and canola oil (GM foods hide everywhere today, often where you least expect them)

▶ Unhealthy fats (processed vegetable oils)

▶ Casein (the protein found in dairy products including milk and cheese)

Keep in mind that inflammation happens when a set of reparative chemicals in the blood are activated due to injury, infection, or even psychological stress. Clearly, inflammation is one of the ways in which the immune system reacts to a threat—with the intention to heal. Since most threats come into contact with our bodies at the level of the gut, and most of our immune system is also located there, chances are that inflammation begins with gut dysfunction. Once upon a time in our history, this response was adaptive, but the reality of our modern lifestyles has left many of us with an inflammatory response that's activated at all times.

One of the most effective ways to heal a dysfunctional immune system—and thyroid gland—is by eliminating sugar and getting blood sugar under control. You read that right: the secret to ending your depression could very well be in stopping the highs and lows (the sugar roller coaster) that are taking place in your bloodstream and, by implication, your brain.[10] And balancing blood sugar chaos may also save you from a diagnosis of panic disorder, generalized anxiety, symptoms associated with ADHD diagnoses, and even bipolar disorder and keep you from relying on medication that can inflict harm on your mind and body.

BLOOD SUGAR BEDLAM

You know the haze that can descend on you with a post-lunch sugar crash, and you've probably experienced the crankiness ("hangriness") of low blood sugar for yourself, if not in your own body then in your child or someone close to you. But blood sugar imbalances can also be chronic, and progressively serious. Insulin resistance, the first stop on the express train to a diabetes diagnosis, is a potentially grave condition—one that's affecting Americans in epic numbers. While diabetes and obesity often share the limelight, prolonged insulin resistance and its partner reactive hypoglycemia, frequently manifest as classical psychiatric symptoms. In many people, their dietary choices—heavy in refined, processed carbs and low in healthy fats—lead to taking psychiatric medications before addressing the blood sugar problems that lie at the root of the problem. And when you consider the hidden impact that ingredients like gluten, artificial sugars, and dairy proteins could be having on the body's immune system *in addition to* the blood sugar issues, it's a double whammy.

Insulin, as you likely already know, is one of the body's most important substances. It's a hormone best known for helping us move carbohydrate-based energy from food into cells for their use. The process by which our cells take in and utilize the vital sugar molecule glucose, the body's primary source of energy, is uniquely complex. Our cells cannot pick up glucose passing by in the bloodstream. They have to transport the molecule with the help of insulin, which is produced by the pancreas. Insulin whisks glucose from the bloodstream into muscle, liver, and especially fat cells, so it can then be used as fuel, or it can be stored as energy in the form of fat.

Normal, healthy cells have no problem responding to insulin. But when cells are relentlessly exposed to high levels of insulin as a result of a persistent spike in glucose—again, typically caused by consuming too many modern carbohydrates—our cells adapt and become "resistant" to the hormone. This triggers the pancreas to pump out more, so now higher levels of insulin are required for glucose to enter cells. But these higher levels also plummet blood sugar, resulting in brain-based panic and bodily discomfort. In fact, many of the words used to describe the sensation of blood sugar hitting rock bottom are synonymous with depression.

As you can imagine, a vicious cycle is set in motion that eventually can culminate in type 2 diabetes. If you're a diabetic, by definition you have high blood sugar because your body cannot transport critical glucose into cells, where it can be safely stored for energy. And if that glucose remains in the blood, it will cause a lot of damage. No wonder the primary morbidity and mortality associated with high blood sugar is the number one form of death in the Western world: heart disease. And as I noted in Chapter 1, it's also no surprise that high blood sugar is one of the biggest risk factors for depression. Women with diabetes are nearly 30 percent more likely to develop depression. In 2015, a study led by a team of scientists at Michigan State and Dankook University in South Korea found that inflammation (as measured by high C-reactive protein) and metabolic disorders like high fasting blood sugar and glycated hemoglobin were extremely predictive of depression in women, much more so than in men.[11]

This might be a tough lesson to learn, and I know because I myself am a recovering sugar addict. But we weren't designed to eat the amounts and types of sugars that we are consuming today, some of which are hidden in seemingly innocuous foods marketed as healthy (such as whole grain, complex carbohydrate cereals, low-fat yogurts, and diet sodas containing artificial sugars). The reaction that takes place in the body in response to this high intake of various forms of sugar is called reactive hypoglycemia, which can masquerade as a number of different symptoms consistent with depression and anxiety.

Here's how it happens in a nutshell: when you eat sugar in an obvious form like a candy bar, or even in a non-obvious form such as bread or pasta made from refined flour, you're going to see an elevation in blood sugar and then a compensatory spike in your insulin levels. And that spike ultimately leads to a crash in your blood sugar and a compensatory cortisol response (responsible for moving sugar out of storage and into the bloodstream), which generates more of the same: craving for more carbs and sugars—a vicious cycle. (Remember: your brain can only last a few minutes without a steady source of fuel. If it has been dependent on sugar rather than the more steady source fat, you are in for a world of hurt when blood sugar crashes!) In this state, you're likely to feel jittery, anxious, headachy, nauseous, irritable, edgy, moody, tired, and foggy. Sound familiar? All of these symptoms can come under a diagnosis of depression and anxiety. And these feelings can last all throughout the day, week, month, contributing to a general sense of unease and agitation that might land you in your doctor's office with her handing you a prescription for an antidepressant.

Additionally, sugar can damage brain cells in areas like the hippocampus that are responsible for orchestrating cortisol supply and demand. But thankfully there's a simple resolution to this, which we'll explore in Chapter 6: eliminating those abusive sugars and refined flours and consuming more high-quality proteins and natural fats, especially at breakfast.

Case in point: Jessica was twenty-three years old when she entered my office complaining of PMS with acne and a pervasive feeling of unease that qualified as textbook depression. She frequently woke up in the middle of the night to snack but wasn't hungry when she dragged herself out of bed in the morning. This little tidbit was enough to tell me that her blood sugar balance was a distant memory. She also mentioned nagging fogginess, low energy, a low libido, and racing heart—all details that further clued me in to her blood sugar mayhem. I immediately put her on a dietary protocol that would stabilize her blood sugar and help her avoid the midnight munchies. Some of her dietary changes included the elimination of sugar and grains, the addition of ghee and coconut oil, and supplementing with L-carnitine and chromium. Within just a few weeks she had lost eight pounds, was sleeping through the night for the first time in four years, had no menstrual complaints by her third cycle, and felt free. The ongoing anxiety that had clouded her days had disappeared.

Remember, You Are in Control

When I lecture on the topics that I covered in this chapter, I often get asked about the role of genetics. While it's true that a person can be more susceptible to conditions like hypothyroidism and diabetes due to hereditary factors stenciled into their DNA, those factors don't have to translate to fate. Even someone whose family patterns puts them at a higher risk for depressive symptoms isn't destined to suffer. Your DNA and how it is expressed is constantly at the mercy of environmental forces (i.e., your lifestyle choices—what you eat, how much stress you carry, the toxicants you encounter, even the thoughts you have). A simple way to understand this is to consider an obese person who loses all the extra weight. She still has the same underlying DNA, but clearly the genes are expressing themselves very differently as a result of a change in the environment involving food choices and exercise regimens. And it works both ways: you can have no genetic risk factors for something like hypothyroidism (or diabetes or obesity or depression for that matter) and still develop these conditions by virtue of your daily habits.

Thyroid dysfunction and blood sugar disorders are just two of the psychiatric pretenders that often go unidentified and unresolved when a person is labeled as depressed; others come from external sources, such as the beauty products you buy and the pills you pop to relieve heartburn. Brain symptoms that become part of a diagnosis of depression are almost always traceable to some combination of dietary incompatibilities and chemical exposures from the environment, including medications and vaccines. In the next chapter, we'll see what sorts of exposures can have an impact on the body that translates into matters of mind, mood, and memory.

CHAPTER 5

Why Body Lotions, Tap Water, and OTC Pain Relievers Should Come with New Warning Labels

*Common Exposures and Drugs
That Can Lead to Depression*

Advil, Lipitor, Prilosec, fluoride, "fragrance," vaccines, and birth control pills have a lot in common: depression

When Monica, a fifty-six-year-old executive at a PR firm, first came to me, her two chief concerns were severe forgetfulness (bad enough to make her wonder if she had early-onset Alzheimer's disease) and feeling depressed. She even harbored thoughts of suicide. Monica hadn't always been like this, and she wanted to get back to her "real" self. In addition to her memory and mood issues, she also suffered from low energy, pervasive pain, dry skin, constipation, and weight gain. Like so many middle-aged women, she was taking a statin for high cholesterol as well as a popular antidepressant. Her primary doctor said that dietary changes could do nothing to help. In my workup, I found that she had what I had—Hashimoto's thyroiditis. I also discovered that she showed early signs of diabetes; her blood sugar was out of control.

Monica never thought anything of her statin use, and her doctor had assured her it was a very safe medication, one of the most commonly prescribed drugs, with millions of people taking them every day. He had not mentioned their potential to cause serious mood and memory problems, among other side effects.

Upon learning about the incriminating data, Monica stopped taking the drug and instead addressed her high cholesterol by addressing her thyroid imbalance, a known cause of cholesterol derailment. Beyond the usual recommendations for cutting out processed foods, I talked to her about eliminating gluten (and the inflammation it causes). Monica also received a natural thyroid hormone (not a synthetic one a doctor would typically prescribe), and within three months her symptoms completely resolved and her blood sugar came into balance. In what seemed like a miracle to her, Monica soon became depression free with healthy cholesterol levels. Not only did her good memory return, but she watched the numbers go down on the weight scale. We then worked on tapering her off of her antidepressant.

While it's common knowledge now that we live in a world where exposure to pollution and synthetic chemicals is an everyday reality, what's not so well understood is the impact chemical exposures have on the female body, which can eventually manifest in cognitive and mental issues. And I'm not just talking about the usual suspects, such as plastics and printer receipts that leach bisphenol A, pesticides in produce, antibiotics in meat products, mercury in fish, or smog in your daily breath. I'm also referring to mind-altering chemicals that we introduce to our bodies through seemingly innocuous medications: birth control pills, statins, acid-reflux drugs like Prilosec and Nexium, and nonsteroidal anti-inflammatories such as ibuprofen (Advil) and naproxen (Aleve).

I've already talked about some of these culprits. Now I'm going to set the record straight on "non-psychiatric" drugs that can trigger symptoms of depression while also revealing common sources of environmental toxins that we can easily limit in our daily lives. We'll start with my three biggest pet peeves—the drugs I work hardest to get patients off of. It's not that challenging, especially compared to coming off of antidepressants, but I still have to make my case when my patients arrive in my office with what they think are sound reasons to stay on their antidepressants. I'll then list a few more problematic drugs that are all too common in people's purses and medicine cabinets today and end with a highly cautionary note about vaccines.

PET PEEVE #1: BIRTH CONTROL

When patients come to me complaining of low libido, low or flat mood, weight gain, hair loss, and cloudy thinking, one of my first questions is: "Are you on the Pill?" When they lament about pre-menstrual irritability, insomnia, tearfulness, bloating, and breast tenderness as a prelude to requesting that I sanction beginning a course of oral contraceptives and perhaps an antidepressant—the one-size-fits-all panacea of psychiatrists and gynecologists nationwide—my response is simply "There's a better way."

I once looked toward birth control as a woman's right, an entitlement for the modern-day gal. It took years before I had a complete reversal of this way of thinking. I started to think about the fact that the Pill puts the burden of preventing an unwanted pregnancy wholly on the woman while dismissing and ignoring a range of side effects from vague and insidious to deadly.

With more than 100 million women around the world using this form of hormonal suppression, I have to wonder how many of them have had any exposure to information about the Pill's subtle disruptions to the system, not to mention the risks of thrombo-embolism (major blood clots), hypertension (high blood pressure), cerebrovascular events, gallstones, and cancer.[1]

As notorious as our hormones are for wreaking havoc, they are what pop us into high gear—they excite us, move us, drive us, and enliven us. The intricate relationships among sex hormones, thyroid hormones, and adrenal hormones are like the magic of 3-D glasses: if you cover one lens, things just don't look as exciting.[2]

When a woman is sitting in my office, I know she is someone who has struggled with mood and anxiety, and the last thing she should be doing is stacking the cards against her recovery with synthetic hormones and the pharmacologic burden they bring. Since the 1960s, there has been controversy around the potential mood effects of oral contraceptives, but more than fifty years of their use has not settled the question.

There is, however, acknowledgment that depression is the most common reason for stopping the Pill. I don't need to be persuaded by studies that demonstrate that women using the Pill are significantly more depressed than a control group of women not on the Pill. I see this phenomena firsthand, most notably in those who begin contraception postpartum.

Although the data pointing to a relationship between the Pill and mood disorders is compromised by poorly done studies, what we can cull from the findings is that oral contraceptives represent a major risk factor for depression and/or related mood disturbance for certain women. Who might these women be? From thirteen prospective trials, it appears that they have a personal or family psychiatric history (though doesn't that include the entire population at this point?), one that has been exacerbated by the experiences of pregnancy/postpartum, premenstrual periods, and being of young age.[3,4] More specifically, women who have premenstrual mood symptoms prior to using the Pill experience more adverse effects with pills that contain lower progestin dosages or triphasic oral contraceptives; women without this history experience more psychiatric side effects with pills that contain higher levels of progestin.

Could these side effects be just coincidence? Could they represent "confounding by indication," or the fact that many women who opt to suppress their cycle already might be prone to depression? It's possible, but so are some of the following important biological insights.

For starters, synthetic hormones like those in combined oral contraceptives that contain estrogen and a progestin increase thyroid and sex hormone–binding globulin (SHBG), effectively decreasing the available testosterone and thyroid hormone in circulation, which can render you of nun-like libido and functionally hypothyroid or depressed, constipated, overweight, cloudy, and with dry skin and hair to boot! A randomized nine-week trial of three forms of the Pill found that they all increased both SHBG, insulin resistance, and markers of inflammation such as C-reactive protein.[5] Another study found that increases in SHBG may persist long after stopping the Pill, contributing to sexual dysfunction/low libido.[6] Incidentally, both industrial chemicals that are ubiquitous in our society such as PCBs, BPA, and phthalates and poor excretion of estrogen as occurs with gut dysbiosis can lead to undesirable states of estrogen dominance. This means the body's estrogen/progesterone balance is off.

Second, oral contraceptives promote oxidative stress. Stress is often defined as the inability to cope with demands, and oxidative stress is a destructive force in the body perpetuated by reactive oxygen species ("free radicals") that outnumber available antioxidant enzymes and factors. One measure of oxidative stress, lipid peroxidation (basically a marker of how rancid the fats in your blood are), was found to be higher in those taking oral contraceptives and improved (not quite to baseline controls) when they were treated with vitamins E and C, known antioxidants.[7]

The third big strike against oral contraceptives is that they deplete vitamins, minerals, and antioxidants.[8] More specifically, they've been acknowledged to deplete vitamin B_6, a cofactor in the production of important neurotransmitters that help regulate mood such as serotonin and gamma-aminobutyric acid (GABA), as well as zinc, selenium, phosphorus, and magnesium.[9] Birth control pill use has also increasingly been shown to be associated with elevated levels of copper (which can cause feelings of overstimulation), iron (which can induce oxidative stress), calcium, and cadmium compared to controls. Given that replacing and correcting these vitamins can be an imperfect effort, perhaps it's best not to mess with them in the first place!

Keep in mind that oral contraceptives are drugs designed for healthy people. So they should be held to a standard of benefit versus risk that is distinct from that of an intervention designed as a treatment. Because so many critical questions have not been asked about what happens when we manipulate the hormonal pathways and feedback loops in the body, we rely on observational research conducted on those already taking the Pill. Unfortunately, this means documenting those who experience serious complications related to the Pill, from heart attacks and strokes to seizures, liver tumors, severe mood swings, and suicide. These include young girls and women prescribed the Pill for acne or irregular periods and those who just want to avoid having an inconvenient period altogether. These dangerous reactions pepper a landscape of flattened mood, libido, personality changes, and autoimmune disease all related to the effects of synthetic estrogen and progesterone (known as progestin) that entail adverse changes to the microbiome, metabolism, and inflammatory pathways.

Who ends up treating these insidious side effects?

You guessed it. Your trusted psychiatrist, with prescription pad in hand.

This is why new data implicating the Pill in brain-based changes may finally usher in research confirming what millions of women around the world have been complaining about for decades: the Pill makes them crazy, makes them depressed, and makes them anxious. It bears repeating that there's just no free lunch with medication treatment, and a risk/benefit analysis is very difficult to accomplish if we don't know what environmental and genetic risks an individual is bringing to the table. If you don't know whether you'll end up depressed or, worse, dying from the Pill, why take that chance? If there is a treatment option that presents minimal to no appreciable risks and some degree of evidence-based benefit, to me this would represent the kinder, gentler road to health. These days, women's lib looks a lot more like a healthy, happy menstrual cycle free from the grips of a prescription.

PET PEEVE #2: STATINS[10]

Better safe than sorry, right? This is the logic that defines the grasp that the pharmaceutical company has on our psyche. Chances are you or someone you know takes a cholesterol-lowering drug such as Crestor, Lipitor, or Zocor. Perhaps your mother, father, brother, or boyfriend take one under the assumption a statin will help prevent a fatal heart attack. Recent guidelines have expanded the pool of potential statin users, so that there are very few of us who seem to be walking around with acceptable levels of sludge clogging our arteries. The new guidelines, released in 2013, added 13 million new people to the pool of candidates for statin treatment.[11] Many of these new patients are in the older population, those sixty to seventy-five years old. It's estimated that almost 80 percent of people in that age group would be recommended to be on a statin based on the new risk-based algorithm. And that new algorithm doesn't only include risk for a cardiovascular event. Statins are now recommended for people who don't have high cholesterol or even a risk for heart disease.

But how did drug companies convince doctors that their patients need these medications, and that they need them now? They are banking (literally) on the fact that you haven't brushed up on statistics in a while.

It turns out that the medical literature performs a common sleight of hand with the popularization of claims around "relative risk reduction," which can make an effect appear meaningful when the "absolute risk reduction" reveals its insignificance. This was eloquently described by Dr. David M. Diamond, a professor of psychology, molecular pharmacology, and physiology at the University of South Florida, and Dr. Uffe Ravnskov, an independent health researcher and an expert in cholesterol and cardiovascular disease. In their 2015 paper for *Expert Review of Clinical Pharmacology,* they show how the benefits of statins have been exaggerated and that their supporters use "statistical deception" to make inflated claims about their effectiveness while minimizing their side effects.[12] As

Diamond and Ravnskov explain, let's say one hundred people are treated with statin medications to benefit one of those people. Statins benefit only about 1 percent of the population, which means that only one out of one hundred people treated with a statin will have one less heart attack. But we don't hear about the 1 percent effect. Instead, statin researchers transform the 1 percent effect using "relative risk," another statistic that creates the appearance that statins benefit 30 to 50 percent of the population. So in this case, the change from a 2 percent to a 1 percent heart attack rate is billed as a 50 percent reduction rather than a 1 percent improvement, *which is what it actually is.*

Maybe this would still qualify as better safe than sorry if these medications weren't some of the most toxic chemicals willfully ingested, with at least three hundred adverse health effects documented to date, including muscle and nerve damage, cancer, liver damage, hormonal chaos, and birth defects to children exposed in utero. Ironically, cholesterol-lowering statins, which are among the most commonly prescribed drugs, are now being touted as a way to reduce overall levels of inflammation. But new research also reveals that statins *may lessen brain function and increase risk for diabetes, heart disease, and depression.* The reason is simple: the body and, especially, the brain need cholesterol to thrive. Reams of scientific data show time and time again that extremely low cholesterol levels are linked to depression, memory loss, and even violence to oneself and others.[13]

Since the 1950s, we've been told that eating fat makes you fat and that avoiding traditional fats (such as butter, animal meats, and eggs) in lieu of industrialized, man-made fat substitutes is highly recommended.[14] Why did we agree to disavow several millennia of instinctive eating in favor of a high-carb and high-sugar diet deficient in this staple?

It started with a misinterpretation of a manipulated study.[15] In 1958, Ancel Keys set out to "prove" a correlation between the consumption of saturated fat (rendered synonymous with animal fat, which is typically high in polyunsaturated and monounsaturated fats) and heart disease. He tabulated the incidence of this multidimensional, chronic medical problem in twenty-two nations. He must have been disappointed by the scattered dots on his graph, so he obscured a couple of them until he found a linear relationship between six of those surveyed.

This study seemed to be the green light that corporate food execs needed to get to work making and distributing hydrogenated butter-like substances and processed vegetable oils. In the wake of this tremendous shift in nutrition from real food to manufactured food, we have suffered ever-escalating rates of chronic inflammatory diseases like diabetes and the very heart disease we were aiming to prevent. But what beyond an overworked pancreas and an irritated vascular system do we have to worry about in this low-fat world?

Here I would recommend that women struggling with hormonal imbalance and mood symptoms listen up, because it turns out that cholesterol is a vital nutrient for brain health, a fact that has gotten lost amid all the fat slamming. Have you noticed that there is an upper limit for cholesterol on your lab results, but no lower limit? This may be related to a gross lack of appreciation for the risks associated with hypocholesterolemia, or abnormally low levels of cholesterol in the blood. Cholesterol performs many vital functions, but we'll focus on three specifically: cell membrane structure and support, hormone synthesis, and vitamin D production.

As my patients' lab results come in, I often note that those with mood symptoms invariably have a fasting cholesterol below 160. Their internists may be impressed and pleased with their low-fat diets, but I'm not. Rather than experiencing reassurance that waxy goo is not clogging up their pipes, I envision floppy, decrepit cell membranes adrift in a hormone-less wasteland.

The cell membrane is an eight-nanometer-thick magical pearly gate where information, nutrients, and cellular messengers are trafficked through protein gates supported by phospholipids and their polyunsaturated fatty acids. Cholesterol and saturated fat provide essential rigidity in balance with other membrane components. Without them, the membrane becomes a porous, dysfunctional swinging gate. Cholesterol also supports the production of bile acids, which are integral to the breakdown and absorption of essential dietary fats. Moreover, cholesterol is an essential fuel for neurons. In fact, 25 percent of the total amount of cholesterol found in the human body is localized in the brain, most of it—up to 70 percent of it—is found in the myelin sheath that coats and insulates the nerves. Put simply, the brain is the most cholesterol-rich organ in the body.[16]

The body also recruits cholesterol to produce pregnenolone, a molecule that's a precursor to sex hormones such as testosterone and estrogen, so without it our reproductive and endocrine systems go awry. Think libido, harmonious menstrual cycle, clear skin, balanced metabolism, and cognition. Additionally, vitamin D, a steroid-like wonder hormone, is produced from cholesterol precursors and its deficiency appears to be correlated with maladies too numerous to mention (but, yes, including depression). The body makes vitamin D from cholesterol in the skin upon exposure to UV rays from the sun. If you were to look at the chemical formula for vitamin D, you'd have a hard time distinguishing it from cholesterol's formula; they look virtually identical.

So it's no surprise, at least to me, that low cholesterol has been linked to suicide and depression, as well as other neurological disorders.[17] In patients hospitalized for depression, bipolar disorder, and anxiety disorder, significantly more patients than controls have been documented to have low plasma cholesterol.[18] When a team at Duke University assessed the correlation between depressive and anxious personality traits and low cholesterol, they found an undeniable connection.[19] Another looking at the Melbourne Women's Midlife Health Project suggested that improved performance on memory testing was achieved with increased total cholesterol in women who were monitored over time.[20]

But the medical industrial complex would have you believe that cholesterol-lowering medications—statins—equate with preventive medicine. This is an area where we really should have held out on a bit. First we need to better understand and challenge some of the assumed mechanisms of heart disease and figure out why there are so many exceptions to the "high cholesterol = mortality" linear model theory.

Contrary to what is demonstrated in studies that support Big Pharma, we have plenty of evidence to show just how bad some of the side effects of statins can be. In an eight-year retrospective study, it was found that intolerable side effects occurred in 20 percent of those treated with statins.[21] The scientific community has also revealed the extent to which statins impact women in particular. In addition to there being a total lack of proof that statins can benefit women, we know that these drugs can cause decreased cognitive function, cataracts, sexual dysfunction, depression, muscle pain, and diabetes. This last side effect—diabetes—took the medical world by storm when the headlines hit in 2012. Published in the *Archives of Internal Medicine,* a Mayo Clinic study found that the risk of new onset diabetes in postmenopausal women was increased by 48 percent.[22] Plain and simple: "Statin medication use in postmenopausal women is associated with an increased risk for DM." And this was no small study—it entailed more than 160,000 women.

So the next time you hear a doctor recommending a cholesterol-lowering intervention, tell him you'll take that 1 percent increased risk and spare yourself cancer, cognitive dysfunction, myopathy, and diabetes. And then go have a three-egg omelet with the yolks. As with birth control pills, statins are pretty easy to come off. With an eye toward minimizing sources of inflammation such as sugar and sugar-like foods, maximizing nutrient-dense whole foods, and running from commercial concoctions, we can help support our innate bodily processes and the myriad interrelated connections that a linear model fails to encompass.

PET PEEVE #3: ACID-REFLUX MEDICATIONS (PROTON-PUMP INHIBITORS)[23]

Think Prilosec, Nexium, Prevacid, and Protonix. If you have to take a pill to avoid indigestion or acid reflux (sometimes called GERD, or gastroesophageal reflux disease), then I ask you: Have you ever wondered if a change in diet could eliminate your condition? Have you ever asked yourself why you're having these symptoms and what's happening with your digestion? Stomach acid is part of our biology; it's critical for triggering digestive enzymes along with an escort called intrinsic factor for vitamin B_{12} absorption and managing local microbial populations. The problem with acid-reflux medications is that they can render you deficient in B_{12}, which can put you on a path to depression. Let me explain.

Vitamin B_{12} is among the most important vitamins when it comes to depression and mental health. Recall the story of the fifty-seven-year-old woman I mentioned earlier who was treated with months of both antipsychotic and antidepressant medications and given two rounds of electroconvulsive therapy before anyone bothered to check her vitamin B_{12} level. Her symptoms were years in the making and included tearfulness, anxiety, movement abnormalities, constipation, lethargy, and eventually perceptual disturbances (hearing her name called) and the ultimate in severe psychiatric pathology: catatonia. Despite being hospitalized, she remained suicidal, depressed, and lethargic. As documented in a profound research paper: "Within two months of identifying her deficiency, and subsequent B_{12} treatment, she reverted to her baseline of fourteen years previous, and remained stable with no additional treatment."[24]

How can vitamin B_{12} be so important? B_{12} supports myelin, the sheath around nerve fibers that allows for nerve impulses to conduct. So when this vitamin is deficient, it's suspected to drive symptoms such as an impaired gait, loss of sensation, as well as signs of dementia and multiple sclerosis. Clinically, B_{12} may be best known for its role in red blood cell production. If you're deficient, you may end up with pernicious anemia. But what about B_{12}'s role in psychiatric symptoms such as depression, anxiety, fatigue, and even psychosis?

Vitamin B_{12}'s role in neuropsychiatric syndromes can best be explained by two basic biological mechanisms:

Methylation

Methylation is the process of taking a single carbon and three hydrogens, known as a methyl group, and applying it to countless critical functions in your body, such as thinking, repairing DNA, turning on and off genes, building and metabolizing neurotransmitters, and producing energy and cell membranes, fighting infections, and getting rid of environmental toxins, to name a few. DNA methylation in particular is the process of marking genes for expression rather than silencing them. Methylation defects, which can be brought on when certain B vitamins are low, are associated with a wide array of conditions, from depression to cancer.

Homocysteine recycling

Vitamin B_{12} is a primary player in the recycling of a potentially toxic compound—homocysteine. In other words, vitamin B_{12} is necessary to keep this troublemaker in check. High homocysteine levels are typically found in depressive patients and those who suffer from depression. High levels are also a huge risk for heart disease and stroke.

So if you become deficient in B_{12}, and digestive imbalance goes unattended, you will likely develop symptoms that will earn you a prescription for an antidepressant, and the medications will start to pile up.

Numerous studies have shown how proton pump inhibitors trigger vitamin B_{12} deficiency. One notable study published in *JAMA* featured a case control evaluation of 25,956 patients on acid-blocking medication, which found that 12 percent of those taking these medications were deficient in B_{12} at a two-year evaluation, and that the higher their daily dose, the stronger the association.[25] The high rate of false negatives in the usual blood test for B_{12} sufficiency (results that say a person is normal when in fact she isn't) leads me to believe that many more of those pill-popping patients were suffering from the effects of an undetected B_{12} deficiency.

And let me reiterate what I called out in Chapter 3: acid-reflux drugs adversely affect the gut flora. A 2014 cohort study examined the diversity of microbes in stool samples of those taking two doses of proton pump inhibitors and found dramatic changes for the worse after even one week of treatment. What this also means is that by interfering with your stomach acid barrier, these drugs can effectively ruin the integrity of your digestive system; not only will the extraction of nutrients be compromised, but you'll experience the negative effects of undigested food fragments passing to the small intestine, where they can spell trouble.

Now let's turn to my other pet peeves, all of which are pretty easy to avoid if you just say no.

(DON'T) "JUST TAKE A TYLENOL"[26]

"Just take a Tylenol."

This might as well be the American mantra. It's the perspective that we have been indoctrinated to adopt—that our bodies are full of annoying symptoms that can be suppressed by drugs. The main ingredient in Tylenol is acetaminophen, which has been used in the United States for more than seventy years. It's considered a benign over-the-counter medication, used reflexively for aches, pains, and fever, and is widely thought of as safe for pregnancy.

A 2015 study, however, has changed how we should view this pain reliever. It documents insidious new concerns about acetaminophen use that can only be called "zombification."[27] According to this new study, Tylenol and all of its generic identical twins need to add one more side effect to the label: it blunts emotions. In the study, done at Ohio State University, participants who took acetaminophen felt less strong emotions when they saw both pleasant and disturbing photos, compared to those who took placebos. Earlier research had shown that acetaminophen works not only on physical pain, but also on psychological pain. This study took those results one step further by showing that acetaminophen also reduces how much users actually feel positive emotions.

The idea that this drug's actions in the body interfere with our emotions and the processing of information—be it positive or negative—is somewhat terrifying, whether you're a grown adult or vulnerable baby in utero or newborn exposed to this drug. It goes against the survival mechanisms we have evolved over millions of years. And it does all this after one dose within one hour! With effective natural pain alternatives and efforts to get to the root cause of chronic pain, now you have one more reason that this tradeoff may not be worth it.

About 23 percent of American adults (about 52 million people) use a medicine containing acetaminophen each week. It's the most common drug ingredient in the United States, found in more than six hundred medicines. If we were to add up the highest estimates of injuries and deaths linked to acetaminophen, it would result in a total of a little over 110,000 incidents annually.[28]

The toxicity of Tylenol likely stems from its depletion of the body's most vital antioxidant, glutathione, which helps to control oxidative damage and inflammation in the body and especially in the brain. This is why N-acetylcysteine, an amino acid precursor that can enhance glutathione production, is used for treatment in emergency rooms. Adding insult to injury, I should add that acetaminophen has been associated with neurodevelopmental problems in offspring exposed during pregnancy. In a large Norwegian study, mothers were surveyed for acetaminophen exposure in weeks seventeen to thirty of gestation and six months postpartum. Children evaluated at three years were found to have dose-related effects from up to twenty-eight days of cumulative acetaminophen exposure. These effects included motor, communication, and behavioral parameters.[29] Data from *JAMA Pediatrics,* also published in 2015, sounded an alarm that eluded media attention, but did not change the recommendations doled out in OB offices around the country. This prospective Danish study found that those women who took acetaminophen during pregnancy were more likely to have children medicated for ADHD by age seven.[30] And in yet another study that emerged in 2015, and which mainstream media did catch wind of, researchers from the UK conducted a systematic review of 1,888 studies to document the adverse events associated with Tylenol.[31] The adverse events reported included deaths as well as toxicity to the heart, GI tract, and kidneys. And there's a reason why liver damage is listed as a side effect, for acetaminophen has long been known to adversely impact the liver—the body's most important detoxification organ.

Perhaps Tylenol was never your thing. But I bet when it comes to relieving everyday aches and pains, you've tried one of acetaminophen's main competitors. Those of you who keep a Costco-size bottle of Motrin, Advil, or Aleve in the bathroom cabinet, read on.

ADVIL AND OTHER NSAIDS (NON-STEROIDAL ANTI-INFLAMMATORY DRUGS)

As with Tylenol, most people think of over-the-counter pain relievers in the NSAID category (such as ibuprofen and naproxen) as a harmless comfort. But you would be wrong to assume these drugs are nontoxic to your body and brain. NSAIDs are among the most commonly used drugs worldwide and are taken by more than 30 million people every day.[32] Available without prescription, NSAIDs are largely used for the treatment of inflammation and fever—all common features of the rheumatic conditions for which they were initially prescribed.

These particular drugs work by reducing the amount of prostaglandins in the body. Prostaglandins are a family of molecules produced by the body's cells that serve important functions: they promote inflammation that is necessary for healing, they support blood clotting functionality, and they protect the stomach's lining from the damaging effects of acid. These last two functions are critical. Because the prostaglandins that defend the stomach and support blood clotting also are reduced, NSAIDs can wreak havoc on that intestinal lining.

The toxicity of NSAIDs to the upper gastrointestinal tract has long been established, hence the number one side effect listed on their packaging: stomach problems including bleeding, stomach upset, and ulcer. And over the past ten years scientists have further determined that these drugs are just as harmful to the lower GI tract. One of the first well-known experiments showing how destructive NSAIDs are to the small intestine was led by Dr. David Y. Graham, head of gastroenterology at Michael DeBakey Medical Center and professor of medicine at Baylor College of Medicine in Houston in 2005.[33] He and his colleagues used a tiny camera to peek inside the small intestines of twenty-one men and women who used NSAIDs daily and twenty people who did not use the drugs. No one had any symptoms of small intestine problems.

What they discovered spoke for itself: 71 percent of the NSAID users had some damage to their small intestines, compared with 10 percent of the nonusers. Five of the NSAID pill-poppers had large erosions or ulcers, a condition not seen in any of the nonusers.

Our gut lining is important, as it keeps the gut contents away from the bloodstream. If its permeability is increased, intestinal contents are allowed to access the immune system and to set off autoimmune and inflammatory processes.[34] More evidence suggests that unbalanced gut bacteria sets the stage for NSAID-induced leaky gut.[35] These changes occur within three to six months. There are limited ways to mitigate these negative effects, which argues for getting to the root of why one is experiencing pain and resolving it through lifestyle change rather than suppressing it with medications that will whack-a-mole their way to new, chronic, and potentially more debilitating symptoms.

A note for women of reproductive age: in 2015 an astonishing study revealed that these drugs inhibit ovulation after just ten days![36] The researchers documented a significant decrease in progesterone, a hormone essential for ovulation, as well as functional cysts in one third of patients. The researchers indicated that use of these drugs could have a harmful effect on fertility and should be used with caution in women wishing to start a family. That fact alone should be enough to convince you to ditch these drugs.

I know what you're thinking: pain happens sometimes, and pain is pain. What are the alternatives other than grinning and bearing it? My top pick: turmeric extract, otherwise known as curcumin. Turmeric, a member of the ginger family that gives curry powder its yellow color, has long been known to have medicinal value. Its active ingredient, curcumin, is now documented in scientific literature to have powerful anti-inflammatory effects—so much so that it's being investigated for addressing a wide variety of ailments, from dementia to depression and pain in general. In fact, recent studies found that turmeric extract can rival NSAIDs for even things like osteoarthritis and pain associated with the menstrual cycle.[37] I'll be recommending supplemental curcumin in Chapter 9. For acute episodes of pain, try 1-2 grams.

FLUORIDE

There are so many scientific studies showing the direct toxic effects of fluoride on your body that it could only demonstrate the power of industrial influence that it's *not* considered a scientific consensus by now. In a large, systematic review funded by the National Institutes of Health and led by Harvard researchers, scientists concluded that children who live in areas with highly fluoridated water have "significantly lower" IQ scores than those who live in low-fluoride areas. Their conclusions, published in 2012, were incontrovertible: "Findings from our meta-analyses of 27 studies published over 22 years suggest an inverse association between high fluoride exposure and children's intelligence. . . . The results suggest that fluoride may be a developmental neurotoxicant that affects brain development at exposures much below those that can cause toxicity in adults . . ."[38]

Although these findings only correlate exposure to fluoride and risk of cognitive disorder in children, we know from other research that fluoride has direct negative effects on thyroid function and disrupts normal cellular activity in all of us regardless of age. And regardless of the evidence against it, fluoride is still added to 70 percent of US public drinking water supplies.

The sordid history of fluoridation reads like a sci-fi novel. Fluoride is out of an era when "valium was prescribed to housewives, feet were X-rayed for shoe size, cigarettes were harmless, and nuclear testing was exciting to watch. We knew less and understood the world differently."[39]

It amazes me that the medical (and dental) communities are so stubbornly resistant to connect the dots when it comes to the skyrocketing increase of cognitive decline in adults and behavioral issues in children (ADD, ADHD, depression and learning disabilities of all kinds). In fact, there have been more than twenty-three human studies and one hundred animal studies linking fluoride to brain damage.[40] Makes you wonder if the powers that be want to keep us a bit dull upstairs. In addition to the adverse effects I've already described, fluoride can also increase the absorption of aluminum and manganese (not a good thing), calcify the pineal gland (your day/night sensor), damage the hippocampus (the brain's memory center), and injure some of the largest neurons in the brain (purkinje cells).[41] And you already know from Chapter 4 that it can cause hypothyroidism.[42] In 2015, new data from the *British Medical Journal* demonstrated that fluoridated water *doubles* the risk of hypothyroidism.[43]

We used to think that the dose made the poison. Now we understand that the picture of risk is far more nuanced, and better encompassed by concepts like the "cocktail effect," which in basic terms means the sum of a given mix of chemicals is much greater—and more potent—than its individual parts. Fluoride isn't prescribed based on weight, nor has any safe level truly been established by anything other than administrative hand-waving. Today, babies fed formula made with tap water can ingest up to 100 percent greater doses than is deemed "acceptable." Fluoride also crosses the placenta and is dosed to your growing fetus as part of a soup of

environmental toxicants. Haven't our babies and children been subjected to enough population-level experimentation?

In Part 2, I'll be asking you to start filtering your water if you
aren't already, and I'll give you strategies for avoiding this toxin in
your daily life.

"FRAGRANCES" AND OTHER EDCS[44]

Wonder why breast cancer rates are skyrocketing and some girls are
entering puberty before age eight?

The offenders are chemicals in the environment that act like
hormones in the body and have complex epigenetic effects. They
aren't called hormone mimickers for nothing, or, more technically,
xenoestrogens. These are not hormones per se, but they are so similar to hormones like estrogen in structure that they bind to hormone receptor sites throughout the body, causing reactions similar
to those that a hormone would. Endocrine-disrupting chemicals
include bisphenol A (BPA), phthalates, flame retardants, pesticides,
and polychlorinated biphenyl compounds (PCBs). For a complete list, go the Environmental Working Group: www.ewg.org/
research/dirty-dozen-list-endocrine-disruptors.

Our love affair with chemicals is getting complicated. We eat
them, breathe them, slather them on our skin. And when we get
sick, we take more of them. A meta-analysis in the *Journal of Hazardous Materials* has reviewed 143,000 peer-reviewed papers to track
the patterns of emergence and decline of toxic chemicals.[45] Shockingly, this study reveals that fourteen years is an average time span
between the onset of initial safety concerns to the height of concern
and appropriate action. Emblematic of this pattern are DDT, perchlorate, 1,4-dioxane, triclosan, nanomaterials, and microplastics,
making their way into the environment and our homes.

The paper explores the hemming and hawing that we do in flagrant dismissal of the precautionary principle, which states simply
"when in doubt, use a safer alternative." We don't always have a

definitive answer to whether a chemical or combination of chemicals causes biological mayhem. Remember, it can take years for studies to gather enough evidence that the government can justify writing new or stricter standards or regulations and even to take dangerous goods off the market. This echoes the seventeen-year lag for scientific data to make its way into our doctor's office. Put simply, we need to take matters into our own hands.

Xenoestrogens are not easy to avoid, and they are on the rise in our environment. They are found in many pesticides, industrial chemicals, cosmetics, toiletries (such as scented body lotions), and plastics. And they find their way into our water supply too. These chemicals don't readily break down into harmless forms. They instead accumulate in the environment and soils, ultimately getting stored in the fat of animals in increasing amounts as you move up the food chain. We also accumulate these chemicals in our bodies, principally in our fat tissue. Sadly, many of these chemicals are discharged into the environment legally, so they are difficult to control or remove. And because they are used in so many products—from plastic toys to foods, cleaning agents, and nonstick coatings on pans to medical supplies—they are impossible to ban.

Some of these estrogen-mimicking chemicals do have a short half-life (the time it takes for a chemical to lose half of its potency), but they continually flow into the environment to fuel persistent high levels. The effect of simultaneous exposures to many estrogen mimickers has concerned doctors and researchers for years. Take, for example, the compound BPA. Most everyone living in America has traces of this chemical in their bodies. First manufactured in 1891, it was used as a synthetic estrogen drug in women and animals during the first half of the twentieth century. BPA was prescribed to treat numerous conditions related to menstruation, menopause, and nausea during pregnancy and for the prevention of miscarriages. It was injected into animals slated for the butcher block to promote growth. Then BPA's cancer-causing effects became known and it was banned for medical use.

BPA's story should have ended there, but chemists at Bayer and General Electric soon discovered that BPA could form a hard, clear plastic called polycarbonate when it was linked together in long chains (polymerized). And this was strong enough to replace steel. By the late 1950s, commercial manufacturers started putting this substance in plastics and it quickly found its way into multiple goods: cars, electronics, food containers, dental sealants, and even cash register receipts.

Though estimates vary, each year more than 6 billion pounds of BPA are produced globally and more than a million pounds of it gets released into the environment. You've probably read media reports about the perils of BPA in everyday plastics. The push for BPA-free plastics in food containers, for example, stems from research that shows how BPA can generate hormonal imbalances in both women and men. These imbalances can lead to myriad health conditions including infertility and cancer as well as mood disorders and depression.[46] But BPA is just one of thousands of chemicals we encounter in daily life. Thankfully, it's increasingly being phased out of commercial products and the food supply thanks to aggressive consumer lobbying, but its replacement, bisphenol S (BPS), is beginning to be studied, and preliminary research shows that it's at least equally as harmful as BPA.[47] And let's not forget about the other xenoestrogens that continually flood our environment.

Since toxins and toxicants can enter the body in a variety of ways, such as through the skin or lungs, and via a number of sources, including food, air, and water, we can reduce some exposures by choosing safer cleaning supplies and skin-care and beauty products, as well as through diet. I'll be helping you do just that in Part 2.

VACCINES

I recently saw a woman—let's call her Rachel—who was discharged from a psychiatric hospital on three meds and treated for about twelve years. She was having relentless panic attacks, up to six per day. We worked with dietary change, and she came back in tears after only a month, reporting that "those were the first thirty days in my adult life that I haven't had a panic attack."

Then, one week later, she got a flu shot. She hadn't yet put on her thinking hat, the one that says "My immunity is within my control and a pharmaceutical product with egg proteins, unidentified viral DNA from this animal tissue, gelatin, polysorbate 80, the carcinogen formaldehyde, the detergent triton X-100, sucrose, resin, the antibiotic gentamycin, and thimerosal/mercury isn't aligned with this perspective."

She has struggled with debilitating autoimmune-driven side effects since that single shot—one that she received without appropriate informed consent at a CVS pharmacy. I have seen this happen to other patients who take antibiotics that are reflexively doled out for minor colds caused by viruses.

According to several studies, depression, stress, and dysbiosis can load the gun while vaccines pull the trigger on prolonged inflammatory responses and adverse reactions.[48] On the other hand, some studies indicate that depression and other psychiatric phenomena may result from vaccination effects.[49] How do you know if you will suffer psychiatric consequences from a routine vaccine such as Gardasil, a booster shot for tetanus, or the annual flu shot? You don't.

Despite acknowledgment of genetic variants and their relevance to vaccine effects from the likes of Dr. Gregory Poland and his team at the Mayo Clinic, this reality has yet to be acknowledged by the purveyors of this one-size-fits-all product.[50] Vaccines were designed before we knew about DNA, viruses that contaminate cells used to produce them (SV40, retroviruses), the microbiome, or how toxic one chemical can be to one person while leaving another unscathed. One-size-fits-all medicine is no longer appropriate, and we just don't know how to determine who might be at risk for adverse effects ranging from psychiatric conditions to death.

In fact, vaccines are the only pharmaceutical product acknowledged to cause injury and death that is nonetheless recommended to all individuals—regardless of personal or family history. Even the most basic vaccinated versus unvaccinated trials have never been conducted, let alone trials for combinations of vaccines routinely administered simultaneously. Most short-duration vaccine trials actually use another vaccine or an aluminum injection as the placebo!

Remember those same pharmaceutical companies that were up to no good in the licensing and marketing of antidepressants? Well, their multibillion-dollar pet is vaccines, and corporations have been indemnified against the failures of these products since 1986 (you can sue Ford motor company for a failed seat belt, but my patient, for example, could not sue the pharmaceutical company responsible for her injury). They have sold you yet another string of tales. This time, that the vaccine science is settled, that they are perfectly safe and effective for everyone.

This is what the average citizen has been taught to believe by the very corporations profiting from this belief system. So, despite this backdrop of corruption, and despite growing evidence of unpredictable vaccine effect without efficacy, outbreaks in even completely vaccinated populations are blamed on "not enough treatment" (despite repeating the shots over and over with "boosters") and more clearly ineffective vaccines are recommended the same way more psych meds are added when the initial one didn't quite cut it.

I have strong opinions about all pharmaceutical interventions (is that obvious?), but I feel most strongly about *true informed consent,* an acknowledgment of known and unknown risks to every individual.

But what about protection from all those nasty bugs just a handshake away? From our discussion thus far, perhaps you can already appreciate that germs cannot be simply seen as the enemy, and that our risk of severe, disabling illness and death are amplified when we sabotage our immune systems with antibiotics, stress, and poor nutrition.

I learned from Dr. Nicholas Gonzalez, a pioneering clinician whom you met in Chapter 3, that reductionist thinking can make for dangerous interventions. He explained:

Perhaps you're familiar with the Keshan's Disease episode in China some years ago, a subject of particular interest to me because it shows so nicely the potentially ludicrous perspective of Western infectious disease experts. The syndrome is characterized by a severe cardiomyopathy, with resultant irregular heart rhythms, sudden death, and progressive congestive heart failure, occurring only in certain provinces in China. Western epidemiologists arrived to sort it all out, discovering it seemed to be "caused" by a variant of Coxsackie virus. Their solution, in typical Western academic fashion, was of course a vaccine against Coxsackie to be administered to all Chinese young and old. However, there was a smart researcher in the group who pointed out that the disease only affected Chinese in certain provinces. If it were more of an infectious problem, one would expect more widespread incidence since these high and low incidence provinces were not geographically isolated (by mountain ranges, etc.). And since China is a fairly homogeneous genetic population, genetics would not seem to play a role.

To their credit, some began to look at the environment, including the soil. In areas in which Keshan's was endemic, the soils were very depleted in selenium, as were the local inhabitants eating the local food. In areas where the disease was absent, the soil and people were selenium replete. It was suggested that instead of a vaccine, the populations in the high Keshan regions be given selenium supplements. This was done and very quickly the disease came under almost total control (without vaccination) just with selenium. Here's a case where a simple nutritional intervention eliminated an endemic deadly problem.

Did you catch that? Far from germ theory saving the day, the incidence of "infection" only arose in the setting of nutrient deficiency requiring less than a milligram of a basic mineral a day. There are many other instances of these sorts of deficiencies in the infectious disease realm, including vitamin A deficiency in measles and vitamin C deficiency in tetanus.

In short, the host matters, the germ less so.

Is it possible that vaccinology has applied a reductionist—one disease, one drug/vaccine—model to an evolutionarily adapted system with built-in complexities we have barely begun to appreciate? Is it possible that we have misunderstood immunity, or are still fundamentally learning about its most basic principles? If we are to accept that billions of years have gone into priming our physiology for interface with microbes, then we must acknowledge that there is more to immunity than simply jacking up antibody levels.

What is sound advice today may not be so sound tomorrow. Add to this that correctly prescribed FDA-approved drugs kill more than 100,000 Americans every year (some say it's closer to 200,000) and that drug companies have paid $30 billion in fines for repeated fraud, and it's no wonder why some folks question "sound public health advice" and want to decide what is best for their own families.[51] Remember how doctors used to recommend smoking? Remember the 60,000 who had to die before Vioxx was pulled from the market—only after the FDA's own scientist blew the whistle on the organization during a congressional hearing? Remember DDT, the "good for me" pesticide?

Never mind that there are looming congressional hearings investigating claims from CDC senior scientist and whistleblower Dr. William Thompson that he and CDC officials omitted data from a study over a decade ago to conceal the link between the MMR vaccine and autism.[52] Or the lawsuits against vaccine giant Merck alleging management and scientists fraudulently concealed that Merck's mumps vaccine is not as effective as claimed.[53] For an annotated reference on the psychobiology of vaccination, see my website, www.kellybroganmd.com/book-resources. Because you are reading this, your compass tells you that the truth may be something to dig for. As Mark Twain said: "It's easier to fool people than to convince them that they are fooled." Make yourself the exception.

PART TWO

NATURAL TREATMENTS FOR WHOLE-BODY WELLNESS

Sometimes you have to get knocked down
lower than you've ever been to stand up taller
than you ever were.
—Unknown

So here you are. Something about your life's circumstances—your physical body, the experience of your health, or maybe even the way you navigate in society and the world at large—has nudged you to seek a helping hand. To mine for information. To explore. You may be afraid or resistant, but there's also a little voice inside that says: *It's time. Enough is enough. Go.*

Now that you have reached this far in the book, do you still believe that you are broken? Do you think it's your destiny to struggle? Do you feel empty and untethered?

I invite you to challenge these beliefs. I hope the first part of the book has gotten you started. Beliefs can change. You hold the power to transform them.

I want you to get excited about vitalism: your body's ability—its native desire—to recalibrate, reset, and recharge. I want to reconnect you to your inner and outer communities, to what food is really all about, to the idea that you're here not merely to survive but to thrive. I want to see you emerge from symptom resolution to a whole new mind-set about wellness, or better yet, to *experience* your renewed wellness directly and daily. And this starts when you take some simple steps to send your body the right signals—the right "wonder drugs."

I'm betting that you are ready to live a mindful life, to stop living in your head and to start connecting to your purpose. To live fully present. Your journey led you here, so there are no regrets, no apologies. Everything that has happened up until now needed to happen so that you would be ready for mental health and wellness.

Release fear and all it prevents you from doing. Instead, cultivate your intuition and combine it with this newly dis-covered knowledge and you will no longer be dependent on any medication, any doctor, or even any system. You'll be in your power.

This is the new medicine. It's a revolutionary paradigm that makes the old one obsolete.

Now let's go forward.

they outnumber our human cells ten to one. This fact is both exciting and empowering because it means we are not condemned by what we have inherited through our family histories or genes. We can change many parameters about ourselves that have a direct effect on our mental and emotional status. Such parameters include not only the state of our microbiome through our food choices and dietary supplements, but also our exposures from the environment, the quality of sleep we get, and the lifestyle habits we maintain—from exercise to deep breathing—to stave off unyielding and enfeebling stress. And all of these parameters in turn can impact how our genes express themselves. Teaching you how to take such proactive steps is the essence of this part of the book. The book ends with a step-by-step four-week plan that aims to relieve depressive symptoms and put out the fire that triggers those symptoms to begin with.

This chapter focuses on my dietary recommendations and explaining why, for instance, it's important to eliminate certain commonly consumed foods from your plate. At the center of my message is the surprising relationship between the food you eat and your body and brain's biochemistry. Food is indeed information. You must move away from the notion that food is just calories for energy ("fuel"), or that food is simply micronutrients and macronutrients ("building blocks"). Much to the contrary, food is a coevolutionary tool for epigenetic expression. In other words, food literally talks to your cells, neurons included, and that results in how your DNA functions. I'll take a look at very new and exciting data about exosomes, for example, tiny packets of information contained in plants such as ginger that can alter how our genes express themselves.

My food plan minimizes modern highly processed foods containing gluten and dairy that trigger an unwanted immune response. It also increases vitally important fats needed for brain health and blood sugar stability and puts a premium on the sourcing of food—eliminating GMOs and carcinogenic, endocrine-disrupting pesticides. You'll rejoice at not having to count calories or worry about portion control. Once you begin to eat in the manner I am prescribing, you'll rarely overeat again and never get to the point of feeling so ravenous that you'll eat just anything. This nutrition protocol will reprogram your body's sense of real hunger and satiety such that you'll be able to effortlessly eat the right amounts of food for you—and you'll know how much is enough based on genuine instinct. Now that's an incredibly powerful place to be at, the place where you no longer have "diet mentality" and can trust your body's innate cues to tell you what, when, and how much to eat.

Dietary change is a powerful if not the most powerful means of beneficially affecting the microbiome and gut-brain signaling. I often fantasize about an inpatient psychiatric ward where organic ancestral foods are served, meditation and relaxation responses are taught, sleep is supported, and exercise is encouraged. I'd love a randomized trial of outcomes as a means of deconstructing the one-ill, one-pill model! The idea that our Western diet causes cognitive impairment, anxiety, and depression is no longer based on anecdotal evidence. Plenty of studies, some of which I've already shared with you, show without a doubt the adverse emotional, cognitive, and inflammatory impact of the Western diet. These studies demonstrate that a diet marked by processed vegetable fats, sugar, preservatives, and a battery of other chemicals may be setting us up for the development of chronic inflammation when we inevitably experience an immune challenge in the form of infection, stress, or even further toxicant exposure. This could even start as early as in utero.[1,2,3] Which is why the greatest form of preventive medicine is to engage in an eating style that avoids typical processed foods—to follow a dietary protocol that honors real food, the way our bodies are evolved to expect it to look, taste, and feel. Such a diet naturally limits inflammatory foods, promotes nutrient density, and controls blood sugar balance.

My dietary recommendations are not only rooted in years of working with patients and watching them transform themselves through this protocol, but I've done my homework enough to know the science working behind it. I will say, however, that nutrition studies generally are limited. It's very difficult, if not impossible, to conduct traditional studies on diets using a randomized, controlled design as is done with drug studies. One reason why such investigations cannot be compared to pharmaceutical studies is that we cannot use a true placebo group to study essential nutrients. We can't deprive people of certain nutrients they need to live just for the purposes of conducting a study. Moreover, foods contain a staggering number of different molecules. If we identify associations between a particular type of food and a health effect, the exact ingredients that produce such an effect are difficult if not impossible to isolate due to the complex composition of foods and potential interactions among nutrients, underlying genetic factors, and other considerations. And there's the practical issue of basing a nutritional study on people's honest recollections of what they ate as well as controlling for their lifestyle (such as exercise habits and smoking cessation) that can factor into their health equation despite diet.

That all said, we have enough evidence to arrive at general guidelines as to the best starting template for an ailing body and mind. Natural treatments that can help you reclaim control of your mind again in unfathomable ways do exist in our food kingdom. Where are they and how do they work? Let's go there now. And in Chapter 10, I'll help you create meal plans based on the recommendations given below.

EAT NATURALLY[4]

Three months after giving birth to my first child, I thought: When I'm done nursing, I'm going back to vegetarianism. I had the competing impulse to cleanse my diet and to postpone restricting my diet until after I was no longer the sole source of my daughter's nutrition. I was compelled by the clear and urgent need to treat animals with compassion and respect, and I felt sufficiently convinced that I could replicate and supplement (with a high degree of accuracy) the missing nutrients. I also believed, as do many, that such a dietary shift represented a "cleaner" and healthier existence. And I was simultaneously learning about the critical role of fatty acids as they applied to mental health, neurology, and conception.

But it was through my exploration of the importance of fats and fat-soluble vitamins that I began to question my assumption that we can get what we need for health, and particularly reproductive and mental health, from a diet low in animal nutrition. I focused my attention on vitamin A (in its usable form), D, and K_2, in addition to B_6 and B_{12}, choline, zinc, and amino acids including methionine. I already understood the importance of these nutrients to mental health, but it was the work of Weston A. Price that convinced me that there might be far wider benefits.[5]

Dr. Price was a dentist who set out on a world tour to answer the question: Why were the children and grandchildren of his patients suffering from worsening dental health and increasingly more common degenerative diseases? In the early 1900s, there were still populations that were untouched by processed food and burgeoning Western conveniences. He rigorously studied the health impacts of various indigenous diets. First, he found that there is no one diet for health and that humans adapted to a variety of diets for a reason. An Inuit never saw a grain and a high Alpine shepherd never saw a whale. Different people were uniquely adapted to different diets. Second, he established shared criteria for a healthy diet among those from traditional cultures and nonindustrialized areas. This was revelatory to me. The following four main points summarize Dr. Price's findings about the features of these diets that sustained healthy populations where conditions like depression just don't exist:

- ▸ No traditional human group followed a vegetarian diet
- ▸ No traditional human group followed a low-fat diet
- ▸ All traditional diets were local, natural, and whole
- ▸ All traditional human groups used some raw food

What's more, Dr. Price noted that traditional cultures make provisions for the health of future generations by providing special nutrient-rich foods for parents-to-be, pregnant women, and growing children. They teach the dietary principles early to their young (not exposing them to Happy Meals and processed foods like the typical American does).

Suffice it to say I was instantly intrigued by this dietary landscape. I had a food awakening. I then took it upon myself to understand how to interpret the food around and available to me—how to view it through a whole foods lens. My mother is northern Italian and an effortless master chef. I was raised on home cooking, and I learned that the modern Italian diet includes both ancestral staples—simple meats, fish, vegetables, and fruits—and postindustrial foods including pasta, bread, and biscotti. In my approach today, I sweep the kitchen clean and start fresh with a variety of ancestral foods— meat, fish, eggs, vegetables of all varieties, nuts, and seeds. Once the mind-bending junk is removed, your native preferences will guide you. Are you someone who craves red meat and if given permission to eat it rejoices? Are fruit and nuts sort of a take it or leave it for you? Do you just love vegetables? Without calorie counting or portion size, over time you will be guided to the diet that complements your nervous system and relieves the burden on your immune and inflammatory response.

Because there is no one diet for everyone, I suggest a template that complements those who struggle with depression, referred to by Dr. Nicholas Gonzalez as "balanced carnivores." Although my thirty-day plan may seem similar to a cookie cutter "Paleo diet," I differ in my perspective on carbohydrates and in my ultimate permissiveness around reintroduction of gluten-free grains and beans. I have found that most women start to flag on a low-carb diet. I have yet to meet a woman on a long-term low-carb diet who is loving life. Back in my self-experimentation days, I spent two months on a carb-restricted diet, kicking starchy veggies, fruit, and grains to the curb. I felt great for two weeks, and not a day after. I felt cloudy, tired, and started obsessing about moisturizer and conditioner.

So I allow for more carbs, which is crucial to a woman's emotional well-being, as long as they're the *right* carbs. I should also add that people often mistake "Paleo" for super-low carb. That's not so. Carbohydrates have been key to human evolution. There's no way we could have developed such big brains had it not been for our access to carbohydrates in addition to high-quality protein. How and why we developed such large brains has been one of the most perplexing subjects in the study of human evolution, but we're finally beginning to understand the answers thanks to new archaeological, anthropological, physiological, anatomical, and genetic data.

In a 2015 study published in *The Quarterly Review of Biology,* Dr. Karen Hardy and her team from the Catalan Institution for Research and Advanced Studies at the Autonomous University of Barcelona explain that carbohydrate consumption, particularly in the form of starch from tubers, seeds, and fruits and nuts, was key to the rapid growth and development of our brains over the last million years.[6] As we learned how to cook and use fire, our genes for producing salivary amylase, the enzyme to break down carbohydrates, became more abundant and expressive. We have many copies of the genes that code for salivary amylase where as other primates have only two copies. This means we have a much greater ability to digest starch than other primates because we can produce more salivary amylase. We don't know exactly when these genes began to multiply in the human code, but science currently suggests it happened in the last one million years. In other words, our consumption of carbs is nothing new. Hardy also points out that our brains use up to 25 percent of the body's energy budget and up to 60 percent of blood glucose. While we can make glucose from other sources, it's not the most efficient way, and low-carb diets are not likely to meet these high glucose demands.

So there you have it. Carbs are good. But again, they must be the right ones—the unprocessed ones. You will become the balanced carnivore that your body wants to be. For the past eight years, I have used a moderate carb ancestral diet in the treatment of depression with astounding results. This diet focuses on tubers as a source of carbohydrate, and, after one month of slate-clearing (microbial shifting), reincorporates gluten-free grains, white potatoes, and even beans (soaked). In addition to providing a form of usable energy, these "cellular starches" (as opposed to flour-based starches, which are acellular) may play an important gut-rehabilitating role as microbiota-accessible carbohydrates or *prebiotics*.

Sugar and flour-based foods can be particularly problematic for those prone to anxiety and depression because of the simultaneous effects on the hormonal, inflammatory, and gut ecology level.

Now it's time to peel back the layers to the core. Here's a distillation of the five main components of a health-promoting, depression-free diet:

Rule #1: Eliminate Processed Food

You've certainly heard this mantra before. But what exactly does this mean? Processed food is, broadly, anything in a package. More specifically, it is typically anything with a long, unpronounceable ingredient list, and even more specifically, it contains processed/hydrogenated vegetable oils, preservatives, dyes, or sugars. Have you ever seen the number of steps required to produce canola oil? It's roughly the equivalent of building a car. Processed food is processed so that it is portable and shelf-stable; it doesn't go bad nearly as fast as fresh whole food. These goals do not overlap with yours. Let's take a closer look at some of the more problematic ingredients.

Refined carbohydrates and flour

The way most people eat flour is bad for our health for (at least) these reasons: it promotes unstable blood sugar, it is made from pesticide-sprayed grains, and/or it is made from allergenic grains. As you know by now, in my practice I focus on the ways in which unstable blood sugar can masquerade as psychiatric conditions. When some people eat foods that spike their blood sugar, such as breads and cereals, their pancreas swoops in to compensate by stimulating the release of insulin at levels that end up plummeting blood sugar. The experience of low blood sugar is one of discomfort and anxiety—jitteriness, nausea, irritability, cloudiness, fatigue—and the short-term antidote is often another blow to the body's balance. Have you ever eaten a bagel in the morning and chased it with a midmorning doughnut or muffin? On my protocol, you'll eliminate all refined carbs and flours. This includes all kinds of chips, pretzels, crackers, cookies, pastries, muffins, scones, buns, breads, pizza dough, cake, doughnuts, candy, energy bars, fried foods, and anything labeled "fat-free" or "low-fat" unless they are naturally this way (ingredients such as water or vinegar).

Allergens

Gluten, soy, and corn have been identified as allergenic foods, and a leading speculation as to how these foods became and are becoming more allergenic is the nature of their processing, genetic modification through either recombinant DNA technology (for soy and corn) or hybridization, a process that is more natural than recombinant genetic modification but nonetheless not without harm. Unlike genetic modification, which splices genes from one organism to another to create a totally new and unnatural form of life (e.g., genes from salmon inserted into those of tomatoes to create cold-resistant tomatoes), hybridization involves cross-pollinating plant species that wouldn't normally cross-pollinate to have a similar effect: the creation of a new species (e.g., seedless watermelons). Whereas some hybridized foods, like the seedless watermelons of the world, may not present a danger, many plants such as wheat have been highly hybridized over the past fifty years to the extent they contain entirely novel proteins.

Such manipulations can render these foods unrecognizable to our immune systems and vehicles of unwelcome information. When digested or partially digested, gluten (as well as processed dairy) creates peptides that, once through the gut barrier, can stimulate the brain and immune system in inflammatory and even mind-altering ways.

Eliminating gluten is easier than you think; just be careful to steer clear of gluten-free packaged goods, which can be as processed and high glycemic as any gluten-filled food. Gluten-free foods that never had gluten to begin with can be fine, but many gluten-free products replace the gluten with other problematic ingredients such as sugar, GMO cornstarch/meal, and soy.

Below is a cheat sheet of where gluten lurks:

GLUTEN

The following grains and starches contain gluten:

barley	kamut	triticale
bulgur	matzo	wheat
couscous	rye	wheat germ
farina	semolina	
graham flour	spelt	

The following grains and starches are gluten-free:

amaranth	millet	sorghum
arrowroot	potatoes (including sweet potatoes)	soy
buckwheat		tapioca
corn	quinoa	teff
	rice	

The following foods often contain gluten:

bacon	beer	bouillon/broth (commercially prepared)
baked beans (canned)	blue cheeses	

breaded foods

cereals

chocolate milk (commercially prepared)

cold cuts

communion wafers

egg substitute

energy bars

flavored coffees and teas

french fries (often dusted with flour before freezing)

fried vegetables/ tempura

fruit fillings and puddings

gravy

hot dogs

ice cream

imitation crab meat

instant hot drinks

ketchup

malt/malt flavoring

malt vinegar

marinades

mayonnaise

meatballs and meatloaf

nondairy creamer

oat bran (unless certified gluten-free)

oats (unless certified gluten-free)

processed cheese (such as Velveeta)

roasted nuts (that have been cooked in oil rather than dry-roasted)

root beer

salad dressings

sausage

seitan

soups

soy sauce and teriyaki sauce

syrups

tabbouleh

trail mix

veggie burgers

wheatgrass

wine coolers

The following ingredients are often code for gluten:

amino peptide complex

caramel color (frequently made from barley)

cyclodextrin

dextrin

fermented grain extract

Hordeum distichon

Hordeum vulgare

hydrolysate

hydrolyzed malt extract

maltodextrin

modified food starch

natural flavoring

phytosphingosine extract

Secale cereale

Triticum aestivum

Triticum vulgare

vegetable protein (HVP)

In addition to eliminating gluten, you will also evict all grains (not including quinoa and buckwheat, which are technically pseudo-grains), corn, soy, and dairy in the first month of the program. Then I'll teach how to bring some of these back into your life if you wish. You won't, however, reintroduce any gluten-containing foods again on this program.

Sugar

It's in almost every packaged food. Seriously. Look for it and you will find it. It may appear under different names—cane sugar, crystalline fructose, high-fructose corn syrup (see box on page 153)—but it's all sugar. The way the body handles fructose and glucose is different (briefly, fructose goes directly to the liver to be processed, whereas glucose is used by every cell as a fundamental energy unit). Processed fructose—fruit sugar that's commonly derived from sugarcane, sugar beets, and corn—is seven times more likely to result in sticky, caramel-like protein/carbohydrate aggregates called glycation end products, which cause oxidative stress and inflammation. Because the liver deals with it (often by creating fatty deposits, for fructose is a lot more fat-producing than glucose), it doesn't have an immediate effect on blood sugar, but large quantities of fructose from unnatural sources have long-term effects. Numerous studies have shown processed fructose to be associated with impaired glucose tolerance, insulin resistance, and hypertension, among dozens of other conditions. And because it disrupts hormones key to regulating our metabolism, diets high in processed fructose can lead to obesity and its metabolic repercussions.

In addition to contributing to the mood and anxiety roller coaster, all forms of sugar cause changes in our cell membranes, arteries, immune system, hormones, and gut. Sugar is pretty much a metabolic nightmare that we just aren't built to tolerate, let alone in the quantities that the average American eats a year—a whopping 164 pounds. If you need a touch of sweetness, use coconut sap sugar, honey, or maple syrup.

SUGAR		
The following terms are code for sugar:		
evaporated cane juice	crystalline fructose	maltodextrin
	fructose	dextrose
corn syrup	sucrose	beet sugar
high-fructose corn syrup	malt	turbinado sugar
	maltose	invert sugar

Warning: breakfast cereals

Don't be fooled by so-called natural cereals. The cereal aisle in your grocery store is one big display of some of the most packaged, processed products around. Recent reports have exposed the dirty secrets behind popular brands, including Kashi. These boxes of "whole-grain goodness" are anything but; they are commonly contaminated with genetically modified ingredients and associated herbicides/pesticides.[7] Most of these cereals also contain gluten, dyes, industry secret flavor enhancers, and myriad sugars. The effect on your body is a setup for abnormal hunger-inducing stimulation, insulin spiking, and cognitive clouding within an hour or two. Throw away your cereal boxes today.

If you can shake off the cultural conditioning of needing to eat a "breakfast" food, and instead just consume regular food—greens, some fish, broth, and so on upon rising—your options will expand exponentially. If you feel like you need something that reminds you of dessert, try my smoothie (page 282); it will keep you satisfied well into the afternoon.

Rule #2: Eat Whole Foods

Once you eliminate processed (bagged, boxed) foods with long ingredient lists, you're left with focusing on pure, whole, simple foods that often don't even come with nutritional labels: fresh fruits and vegetables ("Eat a rainbow every day," including root vegetables), pastured meats, wild fish, eggs, nuts and seeds, and traditional natural fats like those from animals, olives, and coconut (not processed or manufactured fats). Despite what trendy low-carb diet books would have you believe, root vegetables are an important part of this proto-col. Eat yams and squash with olive oil, coconut oil, or grass-fed ghee (clarified butter) to complement the natural sugars and enhance vita-min absorption. Boiling or steaming vegetables is optimal. After the first month, white rice and white potatoes are fine additions; these are powerful "prebiotics," or bacterial foods that we want to save for the period after which we've re-set the body. In what proportion should you be eating these? Let your inner compass guide you.

Note that although fruit contains fructose, it is packed with other critical complementary nutrients. You'll have the freedom to eat fruit, but it does not feature prominently in this diet.

ORGANIC FOODS

Foods that are important to buy organic:[8]

apples	nectarines	lettuce
celery	grapes	kale/collard greens
strawberries	sweet bell peppers	hot peppers
peaches	potatoes	cucumbers
spinach	cherry tomatoes	

Foods that are less so:

onions	sweet peas (frozen)	cabbage
sweet corn	mangoes	papaya
pineapple	eggplant	sweet potatoes
avocado	cantaloupe	grapefruit
asparagus	kiwi	cauliflower

Glyphosate-free foods

The importance of avoiding foods that have come into contact with or been sprayed with glyphosate cannot be overemphasized. Glyphosate, the main ingredient in Roundup, is the most popular weed-killing herbicide used by conventional farmers worldwide. By 2017 it's estimated that American farmers will apply an astounding 1.35 million metric tons of glyphosate to their crops. That's just under 3 billion pounds, an astronomical number difficult to put into perspective. Glyphosate residue is not just a threat to planetary health; it's a major threat to your microbiome and a reminder that harming nature means harming ourselves.[9]

In 2010, after a fourfold increase in reports of birth defects in Argentina since 2002, a lab study was performed that found low doses of glyphosate causes birth defects in frog and chicken embryos. Other studies that followed demonstrated cardiac anomalies, embryonic death, and multiple malformations and are suspected to be related to oxidized vitamin A toxicity caused by glyphosate.

In March 2015, seventeen experts from eleven countries met at the WHO's International Agency for Research on Cancer in France to discuss the cancer-causing effects of organophosphate pesticides and glyphosate in particular, concluding that it is "probably carcinogenic to humans."[10] According to evidence dug up from the archives of the Environmental Protection Agency in the United States, Monsanto has known about the potential of glyphosate to cause cancer in mammals since 1981.[11]

Many of glyphosate's adverse effects are found at very low doses (as low as the parts per trillion range), comparable to levels of pesticide residues found in food and the environment, challenging the notion that there is such a thing as a safe threshold of exposure.[12]

In sum, glyphosate:

▸ Compromises your ability to detoxify toxins
▸ Slaughters beneficial bugs in your intestines, thereby disrupting the balance of your microbiome

▶ Impairs the function of vitamin D, an important player in human physiology and mood regulation

▶ Depletes key minerals including iron, cobalt, molybdenum, and copper

▶ Impairs the synthesis of tryptophan and tyrosine (important amino acids in protein and neurotransmitter production)

▶ Mimics hormones such as estrogen, driving or stimulating the formation of hormone-sensitive cancers

Monsanto has long told us not to worry. But the deleterious effects of DDT, Agent Orange, and PCBs were only acknowledged after decades of accumulated evidence of irreversible danger to human lives. Until this chemical is banned, focus on organic produce, pastured animal foods, and non-GMO-labeled products. We must stand up in protest against this nonconsensual experiment affecting all forms of life on the planet.

Pastured animal products and wild fish
Pastured animal products come from animals that are allowed to roam free, eating their evolutionarily predetermined natural food. Those animals whose lives are channeled into our own should be treated with as much regard for their innate inclinations as possible. We must support the beauty of a sustainable organic farming system, its freedom from petrochemicals and industrial grains, and the myriad benefits that come from humane cultivation of healthy beings. As a starting template, I recommend eating pastured, organic meats: red meat including lamb, pork, and beef three to five times a week; fish and poultry two to three times a week; and eggs daily. For a list of sustainably caught fish that contain the lowest amounts of toxins, visit the Monterey Bay Aquarium's Seafood Watch (www.seafoodwatch.org). In the post-Fukushima world, I tend to gravitate toward Atlantic salmon, sardines, and anchovies.

Don't hesitate to try chicken and beef bone broths, which have traditionally been used in gut-healing protocols. Because our diets are heavily focused on muscle meat consumption, which delivers a high methionine amino acid profile, we lose out on the benefits of consuming bones, skin, tendons, and other connective tissue, as was ancestral practice. These parts are abundant in health-promoting glycine, an amino acid with calming properties that has been shown to help with insomnia, anxiety, joints, hair, and skin. (Tip: Try adding grass-fed gelatin to warm liquids or hydrolyzed collagen to cold liquids; start with one tablespoon and work up to two. It's flavorless.)

Pastured eggs

I love pastured eggs cooked over low heat in ghee. The low heat keeps the egg's fatty acids and nutrients intact. Pastured eggs come from chickens that are allowed to roam free, eating plants and in-sects (what they would normally eat in the wild). If you've ever bought into the belief that eggs are somehow bad for you because of their cholesterol content, the time has come to put this myth to bed. Eggs are among the most wrongly accused foods of our era. The notion that dietary cholesterol, such as saturated fat from beef, converts directly into blood cholesterol is totally false. Science has never been able to connect dietary fats of animal origin and dietary cholesterol to levels of serum cholesterol or risk for coro-nary heart disease. And when scientists try to track a relationship between serum cholesterol and egg consumption, they continually document that cholesterol levels in people who eat few or no eggs are often identical to people who consume lots of eggs.[13] More than 80 percent of the cholesterol in your blood that is measured on your cholesterol test is produced in your own liver, and contrary to what you might think, consuming cholesterol helps keep your body's production of cholesterol in balance.[14]

Eggs are a perfect food, and the yolk is a nutritional gold mine. Whole eggs—yes, yolks included—contain all of the essential amino acids we need to survive, vitamins and minerals, and antioxidants known to protect our eyes. And they can have far-reaching positive effects on our physiology. Not only do they keep us feeling full and satisfied, but they help us control blood sugar. In 2013, researchers at the University of Connecticut showed that people who ate whole eggs daily improved insulin sensitivity and other cardiovascular risk parameters.[15]

You'll see that I recommend lots of eggs on my dietary protocol. Please don't be afraid of them. Changing up breakfast is often the most powerful interventions I make for my patients, so stop eating cereal and start eating eggs! Eating an egg could be the best way to start your day and set the tone for blood sugar balance. There are so many ways to cook eggs—whether you scramble, fry, poach, or boil them or use them as an ingredient in your dishes, eggs are among the most versatile ingredients. Soft-boil a carton of eggs on a Sunday night and you've got breakfast and/or snacks for the week.

Raw dairy

During the core thirty-day program, I'm going to ask that you avoid dairy entirely, including milk, yogurt, cheese, and ice cream. I will ask that you drink only filtered water. Not even tea is allowable, because teas have diuretic effects. When you're drinking tea, you're not drinking water, and adequate hydration is key to proper energy production and cellular function. After the first thirty days, I will then show you how to see if dairy in moderation can work for you. As a gluten cross-reactant containing immune-stimulating proteins such as butyrophilin (associated with multiple sclerosis) and casein, dairy can be a challenge for many struggling with chronic illness.[16] And you might be surprised to learn that readily available dairy is a highly processed food. I invite you to explore the relative benefits of raw dairy (unpasteurized, nonhomogenized) at www.realmilk. com. Raw dairy typically comes from older breeds of cows that do not produce the beta-casein alpha 1 (A1) protein. The A1 protein found in most commercially produced milk, including organic milk, has been found to aggravate depression as well as other neurological conditions such as autism and schizophrenia (it's also been linked to an increased risk of developing heart disease and insulin-dependent diabetes) potentially through its association with an opiate-like compound called BCM7. Pasteurization destroys important bacteria as well as folate and vitamins A, B_6, and C, it inactivates lipase, lactase, and phosphatase (which aids absorption of calcium), oxidizes cholesterol, and damages omega-3 fatty acids and protein.

Another problem with commercial cow's milk is that it imparts exosomes, which can have far-reaching effects. First discovered nearly thirty years ago, exosomes are extremely small sacs that were initially thought to be like garbage cans whose job was to discard unwanted cellular components. But recent evidence has accumulated to indicate that these dumpsters also act as messengers, conveying information to distant tissues.[17] They contain MicroRNAs (miRNAs), a well-defined group of non-coding small RNAs that "talk" to our genes and get them to "talk back" by controlling their expression. In breast milk, these exosomes are charged with supporting infant immunity as a part of the two-person process of supporting infant development. But they can also relay health-damaging information when they come from certain sources. The miRNAs that come from breast milk and vegetables impart health-promoting information, but the ones that are found in cow's milk have the opposite effect, delivering information that can ultimately trigger inflammation.

Nuts and seeds

All types of seeds (including flax) and dry-roasted or raw nuts are good. Note that peanuts are not nuts—they are a legume and should be avoided for reasons I'll give shortly. For nut butters, be sure to buy the ones with the oil sitting on top and no sugar added. Consider soaking and sprouting nuts to minimize enzyme-inhibitors: measure 4 cups of nuts, cover in filtered water, add 1 to 2 tablespoons of unrefined salt, and leave overnight on the counter. Drain and rinse in the morning. To dry them, put them in the oven or a dehydrator at 100 to 150°F until dry. Some companies will do this for you: look for the word *sprouted* on the bag.

Warning: legumes

I advise my patients to avoid legumes entirely for the first month, as they have what could be described as "invisible thorns" called lectins that confuse the immune system and contribute to a wide range of health conditions related to an increase in inflammation.[18] Popular legumes include beans, peas, lentils, and peanuts. In addition to being high in minerals, vitamins, and fiber, they are also high in what's called resistant starch, which is a special type of fiber that can be helpful once the gut flora is better optimized (it "resists" being digested and helps you feel full). Beans are well tolerated by most and, with the exception of peanuts and soy, can be reintroduced. Unfortunately, peanuts are at high risk for mold and soy can inhibit thyroid and pancreatic enzymes. Once you've reintroduced legumes back in your diet, it's best to soak them overnight in filtered water and rinse them before cooking.

Rule #3: Don't Avoid or Restrict Natural Fats

At some point in your life, I bet you tried to avoid fat, thinking it was making you fat, just like you shunned high-cholesterol foods for fear of them gumming up your arteries. Weight-loss companies, advertisers, grocery stores, food manufacturers, and popular books have long sold the idea that we should be on a low-fat, low-cholesterol diet. Indeed, certain types of fat, such as commercially processed fats and oils, are associated with adverse health outcomes. But not so for unmodified, natural fats, as long as they come from animals or plants.

When my patients complain of sugar-driven mood and anxiety fluctuations, depression, insomnia, and low libido, I know that I need to support their brain, hormone, and metabolic functioning with an aggressive infusion of fat. Lest you remain under the spell of Big Food, know that a large analysis published in 2014 echoed previous data in demonstrating yet again that high consumption of saturated fat does not increase risk of coronary artery disease. And let me repeat: there has never been a study linking eggs to heart attacks (quite the contrary).

TWO UNCOMMON BUT HIGHLY THERAPEUTIC INGREDIENTS TO START USING TODAY

Liver powder

Liver is a lost superfood and the best multivitamin money can buy, as it's a unique source of fat-soluble vitamins including pre-formed A, D, K, and E; minerals; usable iron; antioxidants; and B vitamins. Grass-fed liver should be consumed about twice a week; a desiccated liver powder can make that easier. You can incorporate liver powder into soups, stews, or even smoothies with minimal alteration of flavor. Start with 1 tablespoon twice a week.

Resistant Starch

Starch comes in two varieties, one of which is not enzymatically broken down and serves as a source of fiber in the intestines that has the power to produce anti-inflammatory saturated fats. After one month of a no-grain, no-added-sugar, high-natural-fat diet, introducing resistant starch can contribute to beneficial changes in the intestine that contribute to blood sugar balance and metabolism support. The best way to do this is with cooled white potatoes and white rice, as the cooling process increases the resistant starch. Green plantains are another source of resistant starch. And if you're looking for a shortcut, try potato starch: start with one teaspoon daily in food or in water (you can do it as a shot with each meal) and you can work up to four if you don't have gas or bloating.

The polyunsaturated fats, omega-3 fatty acids, have gotten their share of well-deserved positive press because of what fish and fish oil (EPA and DHA) can do to promote anti-inflammatory activity and cell membrane fluidity, and counter the effects of processed vegetable oils in our American diets. They don't act alone, however. It is tempting to assign foods to different fat groups, but many fats work best in concert with others. For example, grass-fed beef is not all saturated fat; it's actually primarily monounsaturated fat. Nonetheless, saturated fats are critical to cell membrane health and a brain that is 60 percent lipid by dry weight.

Let me set the record straight on omega-3s and omega-6s. The American diet is extremely high in processed omega-6 fats, which are found in many commercial vegetable oils, including safflower oil, corn oil, canola oil, sunflower oil, and soybean oil; vegetable oil represents the number one source of fat in the American diet. You may have heard the news that we are eating too many processed omega-6 fats. I'll take that further by adding that the omega-6 fats that we are eating are so distorted that the body cannot even use them. They serve only to disturb cellular processes and leave the body still longing for natural sources of omega-3s and omega-6s. Contrary to even some health-minded nutritional information, omega-6 fats are critical for brain and immune function and should not be villainized in their natural form (such as from nuts and seeds).

Here's where to source the full complement of fats:

▶ Omega-3 and omega-6 (polyunsaturated) fats: cold-water fish, flax oil, macadamia nut oil, grass-fed meat, eggs, nuts, and seeds
▶ Omega-9s (monounsaturated) fats: olive oil, avocado, almonds, eggs, lard (yes, lard)
▶ Saturated fats: red palm oil, animal meats, ghee, dark chocolate, coconut oil (remember, fats help with absorption of fat-soluble vitamins D, A, K, and E)

Use grass-fed ghee (many can tolerate butter after the month) or coconut oil for high-heat cooking and olive oil for the rest. Ghee is butter that is clarified of lactose and casein (which oxidize at high heat), and it's a powerful source of unique fats such as butyrate, conjugated linoleic acid (CLA), and fat-soluble vitamins A, D, and K. Butyrate can be used for energy and to support gut cell integrity, and it can even have anti-inflammatory effects on the brain. In

Indian tradition, ghee is known to have healing properties distinct from butter that are not captured by an analysis of its macronutrients and micronutrients.

Coconut oil is not a bad fat, contrary to what you might think from erroneous and outdated advertising on the ills of saturated fat. It is a primary source of traditional fat throughout the tropics, and its saturated fat content has a unique profile in that it is made up of medium-chain triglycerides. These fats don't require pancreatic enzymes for digestion and are immediately available for energy. Studied for cognition, lipid balance, immune support, and metabolism, this food is a must for improved fat-burning metabolism for mind and body.

Eliminate all premade salad dressings, most of which contain vegetable oils; use olive oil and vinegar (apple cider vinegar and/or lemon are good choices).

You'll find that fat adds delicious flavor to your food. Cook with as many fresh herbs and spices as you like, especially garlic, ginger, and turmeric—all of which have been shown to have mood-lifting properties. Turmeric, for instance, has been studied for its immune-boosting effects, anti-inflammatory effects, liver detoxification powers, and even antidepressant qualities with comparable efficacy to over a dozen different drugs. Be careful about packaged seasonings and condiments that were made at plants that process wheat, were gamma irradiated, or that contain added sugar.

SALT SHAKER

Throw away your Morton's salt! Buy unprocessed sea salt or Himalayan salt. Himalayan salt boasts more than eighty ionized minerals that were encrusted into the earth more than 200 million years ago. Consumption of this salt supports electrolyte balance, hydration, pH balance, and detoxification, and may contribute to bone health, cardiovascular well-being, and even hair and skin radiance.

Rule #4: Go Pro (as in Probiotics)

As I outlined in Part 1, there is now ample animal research and preliminary human trials to support the ability of gut microbes to influence mood and behavior. Numerous studies have also shown that the administration of probiotics can reverse certain psychological disorders. Throughout history, fermented foods have provided probiotic bacteria in the diet. All traditional cultures fermented their foods, lived in and with nature, and ate from it in a way that promoted a now endangered diversity of gut microbes. Evidence suggests that food fermentation dates back more than seven thousand years to wine making in the Middle East. The Chinese were fermenting cabbage six thousand years ago.

Although for centuries civilizations didn't understand the mechanism behind the fermentation process, the health benefits associated with fermented foods were intuited. People have enjoyed one form of fermented food or another long before probiotics became available as supplements from health food stores. In America, you're probably already familiar with sauerkraut (fermented cabbage) and yogurt (fermented milk products). Korean-Americans probably have a jar of kimchi in their refrigerators. This is a popular spicy condiment usually made from cabbage or cucumber that's the national dish of Korea.

Fermentation is the metabolic process of converting carbohydrates, typically sugars, into other molecules—either alcohols and carbon dioxide or organic acids. The reaction requires the presence of yeast, bacteria, or both, and it takes place in the absence of oxygen (hence the original description of the process as "respiration without air"). In the nineteenth century, the Russian scientist Élie Mechnikov revealed how *Lactobacillus* bacteria could be related to health. Considered the father of immunology, Mechnikov predicted many aspects of current immunobiology and was the first to propose the idea that lactic acid bacteria are beneficial to human health. He won the Nobel Prize in Medicine in 1908. His ideas stemmed largely from recognizing a correlation between the health and longevity of Bulgarian peasants and their consumption of fermented milk products. He even went as far as to suggest that "oral administration of cultures of fermentative bacteria would implant the beneficial bacteria in the intestinal tract."[19]

Mechnikov believed that toxic bacteria in the gut contributed to aging and that lactic acid could help prolong life. His daily diet included sour milk and he is credited with coining the phrase *probiotic* to describe beneficial bacteria. His work inspired twentieth-century Japanese microbiologist Minoru Shirota to look into a relationship between bacteria and good intestinal health. Dr. Shirota's studies paved the way for today's colossal market for probiotics.

Lactic acid fermentation in particular is the process by which foods become probiotic, or rich in beneficial bacteria. In this natural chemical reaction, good bacteria convert the sugar molecules in the food into lactic acid, thereby allowing the bacteria to multiply. The by-product—lactic acid—protects the fermented food from being invaded by harmful bacteria because it creates an acidic environment that kills off bad bacteria. Which is why lactic acid fermentation is also used to preserve foods. To make fermented foods today, certain strains of good bacteria such as *Lactobacillus acidophilus* are introduced to the sugar-containing foods to kick-start the process. Yogurt, for instance, is easily made by using a starter culture (strains of live active bacteria) and milk.

In Chapter 9, I'll share details on what to look for in probiotic supplements, but there's no better way to consume a rich array of healthy bacteria than to consume them through wholly natural sources, such as sauerkraut, pickles, kimchi, and other fermented vegetables. My menu ideas will help you begin to incorporate these foods into your diet starting today. Bacteria consumed in this manner are exceptionally bioavailable (easily accepted by the body), and they go to work in numerous ways. They help maintain the integrity of the gut lining; balance the body's pH; serve as natural antibiotics, antivirals, and antifungals; regulate immunity; and control inflammation.[20] In addition, probiotic bacteria suppress the growth and even invasion of potentially pathogenic bacteria by producing antimicrobial substances called bacteriocins. What's more, as these probiotic bacteria metabolize their sources of fuel from your diet, they liberate various nutrients contained in the foods you eat, making them easier to be absorbed. For example, they increase the availability of vitamins A, C, and K. They also tirelessly produce many of the B group vitamins for us.

What continues to impress me is that minimal but repeated exposure to probiotic bacteria is yielding positive clinical outcomes. A new term used in my field for these good bugs is psychobiotics, following studies showing a connection between their consumption and positive psychological outcomes.[21] Every functional medicine psychiatrist like me has case stories of the "probiotic cure"—of a patient with debilitating symptoms, often in the obsessive-compulsive range, whose symptoms vanished completely with dietary change and probiotic supplementation. As a clinician who demands a lot of her patients with regard to lifestyle change from diet to meditation to environmental and psychological detox, I am awed by a study that exacts results with a simple probiotic. A small-sized study, it was nonetheless powered to offer an answer to the question: Can probiotics treat mood? In a well-designed eight-week study that involved placebos, forty patients diagnosed with major depression were split up and randomized to receive *Lactobacillus acidophilus*, *Lactobacillus casei*, and *Bifidobacterium bifidum* or placebo.[22] Without intervening on these fronts, they controlled for diet and exercise. At the end of eight weeks, there was a significant difference in mood. But perhaps more interestingly, blood work revealed significant metabolic changes in those taking the probiotics—decreases in serum insulin levels as well as markers of inflammation compared with the placebo group.

If a drug were capable of such side benefits rather than the seventy-five unintended consequential side effects (some of which may be permanent and disabling), it would most certainly make the *Times* front page.

Another compelling new study has examined probiotics (*Lactobacillus rhamnosus*) as a randomized intervention in the first six months of life and tracked seventy-five infants through thirteen years.[23]

The study was initially designed to study the risks of eczema. The majority of babies in both groups were born vaginally and formula fed, and some had received antibiotics. The results were remarkable: at the age of thirteen, six of the thirty-five children (17.1 percent) were diagnosed with ADHD or Asperger's syndrome; all six of these kids who received diagnoses were not part of the probiotic group. In other words, the kids who were given probiotics were spared these neuropsychiatric disorders. Those who were diagnosed were also found to have lower numbers of healthy *Bifidobacterium* species bacteria in their stool during the first six months of life. These effects are reflected in rodent studies that demonstrate the stress-regulating and behavior-altering effects of probiotic administration to newborns.[24] Research is currently under way to understand the cause-and-effect relationships between probiotics and psychological well-being. It has been suggested that probiotic exposure may not necessarily lead to the growth of good bacteria, but rather it wields its power through influencing vagal nerve signaling and supporting intestinal integrity.

Rule #5: Eat Mindfully

Ever finish a meal and not remember what it tasted like? Are you swallowing bites whole? Do you work during lunch like I do? During the program, you'll be asked to focus on mindfulness techniques for an entire week. You can get started by using your mealtimes to sit and eat mindfully. So many of us eat while performing other tasks or being entertained by a television, smartphone, or computer. A quiet, settled atmosphere promotes ideal digestion and turning on of the parasympathetic nervous system, designed to support this process. Your digestive processes will be compromised if you share your eating time with distractions such as watching TV, checking e-mail, or getting engaged in heated discussions. Enjoying a meal should not be another obligation on your daily to-do list; try approaching it as a time both to relax and to recharge.

Also try to focus on the food itself, savoring its flavors and textures. Sit down, close your eyes, be thankful for your food, and take small, conscious bites. Try holding your fork in the opposite, less dominant hand. This will automatically slow down your eating. And limit your distractions to the people you're eating with. Think of it as a way to honor the gift of food and the greater blessings of life. It's also a wonderful opportunity to downshift a few gears, bring a greater sense of awareness to your food and the act of eating, and get in sync with fellow diners and your environment or just with yourself.

GET YOUR BODY'S SUPPORT STAFF
FROM FOODS FIRST

Detoxifying your body from the assaults it endures daily is a nutrient-dependent process. It dramatically draws on our available reserves of vitamins, minerals, antioxidants, and amino acids. Which is why replenishing the body with these vital ingredients is key, especially those that are inherently anti-inflammatory in nature or are otherwise famously linked to optimal mental health. These include the right balance of zinc, copper, selenium, magnesium, calcium, tyrosine, tryptophan, and vitamins A, C, E, and the B family, including B_{12} and folate. I recommend that my patients get their nutrients primarily from food; supplementation should be individualized based on inflammatory markers, signs of autoimmunity, and serum levels of vitamins (recommended tests are on page 223).

If you eat according to the guidelines in this chapter and use my menu plans (pages 252 to 254) to bring it all together, you'll be setting the stage for a nervous system in balance, and supplementation will be just window dressing.

CHAPTER 7

The Power of Meditation, Sleep, and Exercise

*Three Simple Lifestyle Habits That Can
Enhance Mental Health*

The relaxation response is a shortcut to healing.

A variety of easy exercises can activate ancient healing
mechanisms.

I have a monkey mind. As a mother, wife, physician, writer, educator, and to-do-list-completer, I recommend that anyone enter my mental space with caution. Even if I played none of these roles and was charged with sitting under a palm tree and relaxing, my chattering racket of a mind would follow me there. I'm sure plenty of you can identify with this.

The universality of this condition, however, is what makes the practice of meditation so vital—and so ingrained in all religions and cultures. Meditation is aimed at increasing everyday performance at tasks and cultivating a state of waking relaxation. And there's plenty of science to prove how it works.

Perhaps you will be persuaded, as I was, by some of the compelling literature that suggests that the simple act of breathing and attending to that breath may be a panacea strong enough to replace your current prescription. The same can be said about sleep and exercise—two keys to overall wellness and psychological well-being.

I'm going to start this chapter by making a compelling case for the practice of meditation, but I'm also going to show you that it needn't be performed in a traditional manner by chanting "om" or even concentrating on an object in a dead-silent room while perched on a pillow. There are many practical ways to meditate that can achieve great results without requiring that you spend all day navel gazing. You can start with something as simple as listening to a guided meditation for several minutes a day and working up to twenty minutes twice a day for a therapeutic effect that activates the relaxation nervous system—the one that allows us to "rest and digest"—and as a result eases symptoms and restores the body to an anti-inflammatory state. As I've been emphasizing over and over again, the interconnectedness of your gut, brain, hormonal and immune systems is impossible to unwind. Until we begin to appreciate this complex relationship, we will not be able to prevent or intervene effectively in depression. For true healing and meaningful prevention, take steps every day toward sending your body the message that it is not being attacked, it is not in danger, and it is well nourished, well supported, and calm.[1]

Now that we have come to appreciate the power of genetic expression as more than simply the roughly twenty thousand genes you're born with, we can now harness tools that optimize the "good" and suppress the "bad." And it turns out our inborn DNA interfaces with an exposome, or elements in our environment, and our conscious behavior, dictating exactly how the book of you will actually be written. As you're about to find out, with one fell swoop, how meditation, sleep, and exercise can accomplish what pharmaceutical companies could only dream about.

THE SCIENCE OF MEDITATION

Although the benefits of meditation have been documented anecdotally and scientifically for decades, only recently have we begun to understand its importance in the area of psychiatry. Volumes of data now explain why it works; one reason is that it stimulates the expression of genes that are powerfully anti-inflammatory in nature and helps stabilize blood sugar. We become calm, cool, and collected on a physical level, which also has the effect of turning the volume down on our brains so we're less likely to hear the noise from our usual judgmental and analytical selves. Before we evolved into complex, critically thinking beings, our brains were a bit less complicated. We knew how to find food, water, and socialize, but we would have had a harder time with calculus and intricate planning. But then we grew bigger brains so we could problem-solve better and think more like Einstein (or figure out the algorithm of after-school activities, pickups, and homework). With the yin of this more advanced human brain and a greater capacity to think came the yang of its toll: we lose a connection to stillness, mental space, and vital emptiness. Which is where the practice of meditation comes into play. The practice allows us to be liberated from our analytical selves. In this state, we are still aware of senses, feelings, and thoughts, but without the negativity. It is a neutral state that allows for simply watching and witnessing without fixing.

Among the first studies to emerge on the effects of meditation came out in 2005 when researchers at Harvard's Massachusetts General Hospital published an imaging study; particular areas of the cerebral cortex were shown to be thicker in people who meditated on a regular basis.[2] Since then numerous studies have documented that "thick-brained" people tend to be smarter and have stronger memories.[3] These cortical areas are involved with attention and sensory processing and are used for planning complicated cognitive behaviors. There are studies showing that people who've been meditating throughout their lives maintain their cerebral thickness in certain areas of the cortex that would likely have thinned out otherwise over time. It appears that meditation is truly an exercise for the brain, as if it helps grow stronger muscles in the areas used.

The 2005 study was among the first to show why meditation promotes a relaxed state: the act induces a shift in brain activity from one area of the cortex to another. Specifically, brain waves in the right frontal cortex, which is a stress center, transfer to the calmer left frontal cortex. Such a movement of brain activity to areas associated with relaxation may explain why meditators are calmer and more content after reaching a meditative state.

Researchers out of the Benson-Henry Institute for Mind Body Medicine in Massachusetts, associated with Harvard, have further shed light on the mechanisms of meditation's psychological effects, in particular with regard to the relaxation response, which can be achieved through various forms of meditation, repetitive prayer, yoga, tai chi, breathing exercises, progressive muscle relaxation, biofeedback, guided imagery, and qi gong.[4] One of the reasons why deep breathing, which is often a cornerstone to these practices, is so effective is that it triggers a parasympathetic nerve response rather than a sympathetic nerve response. When you perceive stress, the sympathetic nervous system springs into action, resulting in surges of the stress hormones cortisol and adrenaline. The parasympathetic nervous system, on the other hand, can trigger a relaxation response. Deep breathing is a way of quickly flipping the switch from high to low alert in seconds as your body calms down on many levels. According to Dr. Herbert Benson, the relaxation response is "a physical state of deep rest that changes the physical and emotional responses to stress" and is characterized by:

- ▶ Decreased metabolism
- ▶ Slower heartbeat and muscle relaxation
- ▶ Slower breathing
- ▶ A decrease in blood pressure
- ▶ An increase in a signaling molecule called nitric oxide that dilates arteries

The lymphatic system also benefits mightily from deep breathing. Lymph is a clear fluid filled with immune cells that moves around the body in a series of vessels. It's pivotal to your immune system because it delivers nutrients and collects cellular waste while helping to destroy pathogens. The deeper you breathe, the more active your lymph system is. Unlike your circulatory system, which has a heart to pump blood, the lymphatic system has no integrated pump. It must rely on your breathing and physical movement to push lymphatic fluid around the body.

Forty years of research support the fact that meditation can directly optimize your genetic expression, but only in the past decade have the tools to assess gene-based changes been available.[5] Far from summoning their inner monks, subjects in the studies simply pop in some ear buds and passively listen to a twenty-minute guided meditation. The researchers have quantified the benefits of the relaxation response by assessing gene expression before, after twenty minutes, after eight weeks of practice, and after long-term meditation routines. In a series of stunning papers, they walk us through the anti-inflammatory effects of this intervention. The study of eight-week and long-term meditators demonstrated evidence of positive changes to gene expression as a result of the relaxation response. And it appears that the relationship between gene expression optimization and relaxation response is dose-related: increasing amounts confer increasing benefit. And even after one session beneficial changes were noted. The scientists theorize that the biological events that take place during meditation essentially *prevent the body from translating psychological worry into physical inflammation.* Which helps explain why mindfulness-based meditation practice has been demonstrated in randomized trials to improve depressive symptoms in fibromyalgia and to have lasting antianxiety effects after only eight weeks of group practice. Though more research is needed, this is powerful evidence of the benefits of meditation.[6]

Meditation can help you cope with stressors in your life that persist and prepare you to meet acute challenges with grace. I know this to be true. I've been a devout meditator for years now; the eleven minutes I spend each morning to take in deep breaths helps me prepare for the day's challenges and tame that tedious monkey mind.

Meditation can simply mean stopping for a moment to be fully present to your inhalation and exhalation; it can entail approaching conflict, tension, and stress with an accepting noncombative mindset; or it can involve using new technologies that help you to recalibrate your nervous system. Below I'll outline a few options and show how you can learn these simple techniques. For more ideas and links to updated online resources and videos and audio programs that take you through guided imagery and breathing practices, go to my website, www.kellybroganmd.com.

Through meditation, you remain a quiet observer of your neurotic mind and eventually the chatter that can fuel and aggravate depression starts to fade into the background. This is a vehicle for defining your comfort zones more broadly, appreciating the limitations of your preferences, and recognizing how unrealistic it is to match up the reality of what happens in your external world with your mostly arbitrary expectations. The truth is that in many ways we create our own distress, and when we try to use our minds to resolve that stress, it simply doesn't work.

Practice Deep Breathing

Deep breathing can be done anywhere, anytime. If you've never meditated before, a deep breathing practice twice daily will get you started and give you a foundation for working up to more advanced techniques.

Basic deep breathing: Sit comfortably in a chair or on the floor. Close your eyes and make sure your body is relaxed, releasing all the tension in your neck, arms, legs, and back. Inhale through your nose for as long as you can, feeling your diaphragm and abdomen rise as your stomach moves outward. Sip in a little more air when you think you've reached the top of your lungs. Slowly exhale to a count of twenty, pushing every breath of air from your lungs. Continue for at least five rounds of deep breaths.

Single-sided deep breathing: One variation on deep breathing is the left-nostril breathing technique, one of my favorites from my kundalini yoga practice (more on this coming up). Left-nostril breathing activates the ida nerve ending in the left nostril, which relates to calmness and relaxation. This kind of breathing is associated with the moon energy, which is changeable, feminine, yin, giving, and cooling. Breathing through the left nostril for five minutes can calm you and lower your blood pressure. Here's how to do it:

Sit comfortably crossed-legged with a straight spine (easy pose). Close your right nostril with your right thumb while your other fingers are stretched straight up as antennas. Your left hand can rest on your left knee. Close your eyes and concentrate at the space between your eyebrows, which is referred to as the third eye. Begin to breathe long and deep only through your left nostril. Continue for three minutes.

Summon Feelings of Gratitude

For twenty years the HeartMath Institute has played a vital role in providing individuals with tools for the implementation of mind-body resonance. Their research uses heart rate variability, or the beat-to-beat changes that influence heart rhythms, to assess the synchronicity between the brain and the heart. As it turns out, summoning up a feeling of gratitude—focusing on specific events, people, and experiences that you appreciate and that bring you joy—while breathing in a paced manner (typically six counts in and six counts out), can flip heart rate variability into the most optimal patterns associated with calm relaxation and peak mental performance. They have validated the effects on ADHD, hypertension, and anxiety with double blind, placebo-controlled, randomized trials.

From the High Tech to Low Tech

Biofeedback devices such as the emWave (see the Resources page on my website) and Muse can help improve progress toward toning that parasympathetic nervous system. Historically people have used biofeedback methods to control muscle tension, skin temperature, and heart rate. Biofeedback sessions entail the attachment of electrical sensors to different parts of your body to monitor your body's physiological state, such as brain waves, skin temperature, and muscle tension. The information gathered is then sent back to you via cues such as visual scenes, sounds, or lights. The goal of the feedback is to teach you to change or control your body's physiological reactions by shifting your thoughts, emotions, or behavior. In turn, this can help the condition you are targeting, from headaches to chronic pain and depression. Biofeedback can essentially reprogram how your body responds to stimuli and perceives pain or negativity.

Many physical therapy clinics, medical centers, and hospitals offer biofeedback training, but a growing number of devices and programs are available for home use. Some of these are handheld portable devices, while others connect to your computer. Try different devices until you find one that works for you. And if biofeedback isn't for you, then rest assured that liberating yourself from the day-to-day perceptions of negativity, overwhelm, and loss may be far less complicated.

One of my favorite books on the subject of how to free ourselves from the effects of stress is *The Untethered Soul* by Michael Singer.[7] Singer makes the bold assertion that happiness and freedom are the result of cultivating "witness consciousness," a state of willfully observing one's own mind, emotions, and behaviors rather than feeling that you *are* these things.

He argues that focus and awareness are what makes disturbances real—a hammer falls on your toe and your awareness moves there, then you hear a bang and your awareness moves there. He implores the reader to experience pain as energy passing through before the eye of consciousness and tasks us with the imperative to relax and release, stay centered, and resist the pull to engage in a reactionary way. Let the parade of thoughts and emotions pass by without running along with it to see where it's going. You remain a quiet

observer of your neurotic mind and eventually the chatter starts to go quiet.

This is a means of defining our comfort zones more broadly, appreciating the limitations of our preferences, and the impossibility of matching up our external world with our arbitrary internal definitions of what should be. I particularly love Singer's analogy of sitting by a river noting a swirl in the water. You could try to frantically smooth out the surface of the water, or you could reach in to pluck the rock out, only to notice that it is your other hand holding it there. In many ways we create our own distress, and then we try to use our brains and emotions to resolve that stress. It just doesn't work.

Here are some basic steps toward developing witness consciousness:

1. Notice and acknowledge your discomfort.
2. Relax and release it no matter how urgent it feels. Let the energy pass through you before you attempt to fix anything.
3. Imagine sitting up tall, in a mental place where you can watch your thoughts, emotions, and behavior with a detached compassion.
4. Then ground yourself. Connect to the present moment—feel the earth under your feet, smell the air, imagine roots growing into the earth from your spine.

This isn't an exercise done for mastery, so do it in a spirit of non-judgment. Engaging this practice is a decision that you make every time you feel disturbed inside; the practical rewards are incalculable.

Try Kundalini Yoga

After doing sweat-inducing vinyasa yoga for more than twenty years, my first experiences with kundalini yoga left me confused and sore. At first I didn't get this style of bizarre yoga with its chanting, seventies-style songs, and repetitive movements that felt like all pain, no gain. But now I'm a card-carrying devotee of kundalini,

which is considered the most comprehensive of yoga traditions, combining meditation, mantra, physical exercises, and breathing techniques. In the summer of 2015 I took my two young daughters on a kundalini retreat for a week so they'd be exposed to the power of this practice early in life. I redoubled my commitment to what the practice has to offer and began my own teacher training journey. It's a method of harnessing your own power, getting out of your own way, and bringing the experience of joy into your life. Sounds good, right?

It helps to think of kundalini yoga as simply a technology to harness your *shakti,* or innate primal creative energy. It holds the promise for bliss and even enlightenment, and it accomplishes these transformative leaps through one- to eleven- (and longer) minute *kriyas* (meditation exercises) that use breath and movement to unearth and help release subconscious negative patterns ingrained in us like computer programs. These are achievements that would otherwise take years and years of psychotherapy and personal work, and sometimes they can be actualized in the space of one practice.

What appeals to my more pragmatic sensibilities is that kundalini yoga is goal oriented.[8] Each kriya is for a specific purpose, and they have been handed down with great care from ancient times and crafted for outcomes in real time. The mantras are for the purpose of cultivating vibrational effects in the brain and nervous system. The breath is for accessing the nervous system in ways that we otherwise cannot. And the movements complement this effort to bring parasympathetic and sympathetic nervous systems into balance while also pushing you into a space of discomfort—a space where energies shift and lasting changes occur. It is the art of playing your body like an instrument. It can be harder than it looks, and what's hard for me may not be hard for you. You can expect the unexpected.

So many of my patients suffer from a feeling of purposelessness, a lack of vitality, and an absence of connectedness to their own energetic reserves. Those reserves that are summoned when you are so

tired that all you can think about is your pillow, and then you find out you just won the lottery and you're bouncing off the walls. That energy was in there waiting the whole time.

Because I can't help but anchor my interests in data, I was pleased to find a small but compelling stack of literature on kundalini including a recent article that compared measures of heart rate variability (HRV) in two different types of meditation. The authors describe the importance of this measure: "The human heartbeat is one of the important examples of complex physiologic fluctuations. The neural control of the cardiovascular system exhibits the complex nonlinear behavior. One form of nonlinear behavior is the continual interaction between the sympathetic and parasympathetic nervous activities to control the spontaneous beat to beat dynamics of heart rate."[9]

In 1999, the Research Group for Mind–Body Dynamics at UC San Diego published a randomized, controlled trial of kundalini versus mindfulness meditation, demonstrating that kundalini was the most effective treatment of all available modalities for obsessive compulsive anxiety symptoms, with a 15-month improvement of 71 percent. Another wonderful paper authored by the same group in 2004 describes specific kundalini techniques for certain psychiatric conditions ranging from anxiety to addiction.[10] Here is one that the author recommends for fighting brain fatigue:

Part 1. Sit with a straight spine with your elbows bent and your upper arms near your rib cage. Your forearms point straight out in front of your body, parallel to the floor. The right palm faces downward and the left palm faces upward. Breathing through your nose, inhale and exhale in eight equal parts. On each part or stroke of the breath, alternately move your hands up and down, with one hand moving up as the other hand moves down. The movement of the hands is slight, 6 to 8 inches, as if you are bouncing a ball. Breathe powerfully. Continue for 3 minutes and then change the hand positions so that the left palm faces downward and the right palm faces upward. Continue for another 3 minutes, then reverse the hand position again for the last 3 minutes for a total time of 9 minutes.

Part 2. Stop the movement and hold the position. Close your

eyes and focus on the center of your chin and begin slow and deep breathing through the nose. Keep your body perfectly still so it can heal itself. Keep your mind quiet, stilling your thoughts. Continue for 5 ½ minutes.

To finish, inhale deeply, hold your breath, make your hands into fists and press them firmly against your chest for 15 seconds, then exhale and release. Inhale deeply again and hold your breath, this time pressing both fists against your navel point for 15 seconds, then exhale. Inhale again, hold your breath, and bend your elbows, bringing your fists near your shoulders, and press your arms firmly against your rib cage for 15 seconds, then exhale. Now relax. This exercise balances the diaphragm and fights brain fatigue. It renews the blood supply to the brain and moves the fluid in the spine. It also is believed to benefit the liver, navel point, spleen, and lymphatic system.

So if optimizing your consciousness and feeling extremely alive again sounds appealing to you, go ahead, give kundalini yoga a whirl. It may be the most productive decision you've ever made! You can go to www.spiritvoyage.com to find videos of the practice's various techniques to help guide you. Don't hesitate to check out local studios in your neighborhood that teach kundalini yoga; they are more common than you might think. And check out the Kundalini Research Institute at www.kundaliniresearchinstitute.org.

Integrating these philosophies, practices, and movement-based routines into your life may do more than support longevity and optimal health. It may reverse chronic disease, eliminate the need for medications, and, most important, confer a greater sense of life satisfaction, happiness, and freedom to be here in the present, where the wonder of this never-before-existent moment is unfolding before you.

This chapter wouldn't be complete without a nod to two other powerful habits to maintain in the name of mental health and wellness: restful, regular sleep and sweat-inducing exercise. Many of us have a love-hate relationship with sleep and exercise. But they are essential to vitality. We are built to move and then rest. The

science behind sleep and exercise today is truly breathtaking. Scientists are finally unraveling the mystery behind the value of sleep and exercise in supporting not just the body's hormonal balance and underlying biological machinery, but in supporting the body's genetic expression—all of which in turn help prevent depression and sustain emotional balance and mental well-being.

THE SORCERY OF SLEEP

Sleep medicine barely existed a few generations ago, but today it's a highly respected field of study that continues to clue us in to the power of sleep in maintaining health and mental wellness. The amount and quality of sleep you get has an astonishing impact on every system in your body. Sleep is not a state of inactivity or a zone in which your body momentarily presses the pause button. It is a necessary phase of profound regeneration. Indeed, billions of molecular tasks go on during sleep at the cellular level to ensure that you can live another day. Clearly, a bad night's sleep or even pulling an all-nighter won't kill you, but prolonged sleep deprivation can have serious consequences, including depression.

Entire books have been written about the proof of sleep's profound role in our lives, with laboratory and clinical studies to boot. Sufficient sleep keeps you sharp, creative, and able to process information in an instant. Studies have convincingly proven that sleep habits ultimately lord over everything about you—how hungry you feel and how much you eat, how efficiently you metabolize that food, how strong your immune system is, how insightful you can be, how well you can cope with stress, and how well you can remember things.[11] Sleeping longer or shorter than seven to eight hours in a twenty-four-hour period has been shown to be associated with a spectrum of health challenges, from cardiovascular disease and diabetes to automobile and workplace accidents, learning and memory problems, weight gain, and, yes, depression and excess mortality. Banking six or less hours for just one night reduces

daytime alertness in most people by about a third, and can even impair your ability to operate machinery and perform basic bodily functions in the way that alcohol can.[12]

One aspect of sleep that is underappreciated but has a large impact on our sense of well-being is its control of our hormonal cycles. Each one of us, men included, harbors an internal biological clock called a circadian rhythm defined by the pattern of recurring activity associated with the environmental cycles of day and night. These are rhythms that repeat roughly every twenty-four hours, and they include our sleep-wake cycle, the shifts of hormones, and the rise and fall of body temperature. When your rhythm is not synchronized properly with the twenty-four-hour solar day, you won't feel 100 percent. If you've traveled across time zones and experienced jet lag, then you know—often painfully—what it means to have a disrupted circadian rhythm.

Put simply, your circadian rhythm hinges on your sleep habits. In fact, a healthy rhythm commands normal hormonal secretion patterns, from those associated with hunger cues to those that relate to stress and cellular recovery. Our chief appetite hormones leptin and ghrelin, for example, orchestrate the stop and go of our eating patterns. Ghrelin tells us we need to eat, and leptin says we've had enough. The science that has made these digestive hormones so popular lately is breathtaking: we now have data to demonstrate that inadequate sleep creates an imbalance of both hormones, which in turn adversely affects hunger and appetite. In one well-cited study, when people slept just four hours a night for two consecutive nights, they experienced a 24 percent increase in hunger and gravitated toward high-calorie treats, salty snacks, and starchy foods.[13] This is probably due to the body's search for a quick energy fix in the form of carbs, which are all too easy to find in the processed, refined varieties.

Cortisol, another hormone, should peak in the morning and wane throughout the day. Levels of this stress- and immune-regulating hormone should be lowest after 11 p.m. when melatonin levels go up. The pineal gland secretes melatonin, and it is

also susceptible to accumulation of aluminum (from sources including vaccines, baking soda, deodorant, and cookware) as well as fluoride (from toothpaste and tap water, as well as some medications).[14] This is a potent antioxidant hormone that signals sleep; for millions of years it alerted your brain that it's dark outside, ultimately helping to regulate your circadian rhythm. Once released, it slows your body down, lowering blood pressure and, in turn, core body temperature so you're ready for sleep. Increasing levels of melatonin facilitate deep sleep, which helps maintain healthy levels of important hormones like growth hormone, thyroid hormone, and sex hormones.

As a highly ritualized behavior, sleep also exemplifies the complexity of physiologic processes that feel beyond our control. Sleep onset involves a parasympathetic nervous system transition, a shift that is impossible to will with our cognitive minds, as 25 percent of Americans struggling with insomnia could tell you.

These days, the emergency calls I get from patients tend to be from those suffering from psychotropic-withdrawal-induced insomnia. Otherwise balanced, rational women are rendered near psychotic by the trauma of insomnia and disrupted sleep cycles. Their bodies and minds have "forgotten" how to do it. It turns out that one of the many poorly elucidated lasting effects of antidepressants is their interference with normal sleep patterns. As articulated by Drs. Andrew Winokur and Nicholas Demartinis for *Psychiatric Times,* ". . . class effects of SSRI therapy appear to include increased sleep onset latency and/or an increased number of awakenings and arousals, leading to an overall decrease in sleep efficiency. Virtually all of the SSRIs examined have been noted to suppress REM sleep. Clinically, reports of a change in the frequency, intensity, and content of dreaming can be associated with SSRIs, as well as the occurrence of these symptoms on discontinuation."[15]

To understand the significance of this, a brief review of normal sleep physiology is in order.[16] Sleep occurs in two major phases: non-rapid eye movement (NREM) and REM sleep. NREM sleep is further divided into stages 1 to 4, with stages 3 and 4 representing slow-wave sleep. Sleep itself is a continuous progression from wake-fulness to NREM sleep to REM sleep. Over the course of a night, four to six cycles of NREM to REM sleep occur, each lasting 80 to 110 minutes, with slow-wave sleep predominating in the early part of the night.

As I've mentioned earlier, during normal physiological sleep, blood levels of cortisol, norepinephrine, and epinephrine drop while growth factors such as growth hormone, prolactin, and melatonin increase. Nocturnal shifts in cortisol result in increased immune cell activity at night. Sleep, particularly slow-wave sleep, supports adaptive immunity, the memory defense that works in concert with the frontline innate immune system. By activating two response systems, the fight-or-flight adrenaline-pumping system and the stress-response hormonal system, or HPA axis, lost sleep can skew immunity function.

Studies have shown that nocturnal sleep primes inflammatory signaling and lost sleep results in daytime inflammation. Women appear to be more susceptible, with those sleeping fewer than eight hours measuring higher levels of inflammatory markers in their blood work. When sleep loss is extended beyond a single night to four days or beyond, inflammation becomes dysregulated. Interestingly, daytime naps appear to compensate for this adverse effect.

If you've ever noticed that you get sick more often when you're sleep deprived, now you know why: sleep disruption can leave you more vulnerable to infection. Each of us brings our inflammatory and immune patterns to our sleep integrity, which then further influences immunity and inflammation.

New science is showing that there's a bidirectional relationship between insomnia, depression, and inflammation such that insomnia *predicts* depression risk by up to fourteenfold after a year.[17] And no doubt the shared pathway is inflammation. Inflammation itself, from sources like infection, food antigens, stress, and toxicant exposure, has also been shown to lead to insomnia. So you can see how a vicious cycle can become established—lack of proper sleep triggers inflammation and inflammation supports more disrupted sleep.

Now that you appreciate the role of sleep in optimal immune and inflammatory functioning, how can you maximize your experience of sleep and free yourself from insomnia? Sleep is a behavioral act that can be reprogrammed and supported. Let me give you some ideas, now, and I'll go into them again during week four of the program when you focus on sleep habits. By then you will have already made changes to your diet that will in turn support restful sleep.

- **Know your number.** Contrary to popular wisdom there's no one-size-fits-all magic number of hours the body requires to sleep. Everyone has different sleep needs. Find out how much you need by determining an optimal wake-up time and then going to bed eight to nine hours before for a week until you wake up before your alarm. Be strict about going to bed and getting up at the same time daily, 365 days a year. Despite what many people attempt to do, shifting your sleep habits on the weekends to catch up can sabotage a healthy circadian rhythm.
- **Unplug to recharge.** Set aside at least thirty minutes before bedtime to unwind and prepare for sleep. Disconnect from stimulating activities (such as work, being on the computer, or texting) and cue the body that it's time for rest. Try a warm Epsom salt bath for the calming effects of magnesium. Listen to soothing music or read. Do some deep breathing exercises before lying down.
- **Tea time.** Drink a calming tea like valerian or chamomile with a tablespoon of gelatin, a food-based powder that's naturally high in calming glycine, which has been studied to aid insomnia.
- **Prioritize a premidnight bedtime.** Because the hours of sleep before midnight are the most rejuvenating of the night, it's critical to be in bed before then, ideally by 10 p.m., to capture the slow-wave sleep that occurs in the early part of the night.

▶ **Minimize blue light from electronics.** Power gadgets down after dusk or use apps like f.lux for your computer screens and use amber-colored lights to replicate the firelight that may be more familiar to our ancestrally programmed brains. Get yourself a pair of glasses that filter out blue light (try www.lowbluelights.com). This intervention is based on the discovery that all light, whether natural sunlight in origin or artificial from lightbulbs, TV screens, computers, smart phone screens, and so on contains a blue wavelength that is most commonly invisible to the eye. This particular light wave-length interferes with melatonin production and stimulates the alert centers in the brain as a survival benefit to keep us awake and aware in daylight. Like any daytime creature, our circadian rhythms dictate that we should be alert during daylight and sleepy at night, when under natural conditions with the setting of the sun the stimulating blue light wavelength disappears. But we creative humans with our synthetic lights and electronic devices expose our brains to an ongoing barrage of blue wave-length light that keeps us in an unnatural state of vigilance in preparation for activity, even late into the night. An outcome of disrupted sleep cycles and chronic insomnia often follows.

▶ **Flip the switch.** Turn off your Wi-Fi and sleep with your cell phone more than six feet from your bed and/or put it in airplane mode. Consider EMF mitigators and Earthing sheets (see the Resources page on my website).

▶ **Go dark.** Use a sleep mask and blackout shades (try a sound machine too if you like). Keep your bedroom clean and cool.

▶ **Do not disturb.** Reserve the bedroom for sleep and sex, and leave the bed if you are struggling to preserve behavioral condi-tioning around time spent there. If you can't get to sleep within twenty minutes, get out of bed and find a place that's comfy with dim lighting and no distractions (no e-mail, TV, or other electronics). Sit comfortably, read, or do some breathing exercises. After twenty minutes or so, go back to bed and see what happens when you're more relaxed. Repeat once or twice if necessary.

▶ **Pop the right pills.** Homeopathy gives us some additional tools. My top five picks:

> Nux Vomica 30C for tension and feeling overworked
> Ignatia Amara for feelings of distress and emotionality around insomnia
> Kali Phosphoricum 30C for nervous fatigue (mental fatigue from demands)
> Ambra Grisea 30C for sleepiness that disappears when you lay down
> Arsenicum Album 30C for waking with anxiety between 1 and 3 a.m.

▶ **Try botanicals noted to help with sleep.** These include magnolia, passionflower, valerian, ashwagandha, and even orally ingested lavender oil, which has shown comparable efficacy to benzodiazepines. These herbs often are found together in sleep formulas and can be taken dried in capsules or as tinctures.

▶ **Get grounded.** Offset the effects of our shoe-wearing, electrical lives by sleeping on a grounding pad (Earthing mat) that stabilizes bioelectrical circuitry.[18]

Sleep is one of the ways we engage our connection to the elements, sun, moon, and circadian mapping of our physiology and psychology. The trouble is that sleep problems are often the first manifestation of ill health. It's also a symptom that perpetuates further development of chronic disease. Rather than suppressing this symptom in a whack-a-mole fashion, investigating root causes is essential. With tens of millions of prescriptions for sleep medications written each year, one would think hypnotics like Ambien are a miracle cure rather than a highly morbid and addictive chemical that improves sleep time by only less than fifteen minutes while increasing the risk of death by fivefold![19] Amazingly, one theory about why these medications are perceived to be effective is because they generate amnesia for the experiencing of not sleeping and waking during the night. Take the opportunity to send your body a signal of safety through movement, time outside, a nutrient-dense whole-food diet, environmental detox, and relaxation. You'll be doing all of that on the program so you can welcome sweet dreams.

The more exercise you get, the better your sleep will be. In fact, a 2012 review of one of the most underappreciated benefits of exercise put it perfectly: "Is Exercise an Alternative Treatment for Chronic Insomnia?"[20] Indeed, it is. And it's also a well-documented treatment for depression.

NATURE'S ANTIDEPRESSANT: EXERCISE

I'll admit it, I once hated exercise. Maybe it was decades of accumulated damage from a high-sugar diet and everyday chemical exposures. Maybe I was just "too busy." Maybe I wasn't convinced it really mattered because I had always been thin. But today I view exercise as one of the pillars of radical change—one of the behaviors that we can expect to yield much more than the sum of its parts. We are designed to move, to sweat, and to commune with our physical selves in this active way.

I know that I'm not the first to tell you that exercise is an antidote for almost everything that ails us. It improves digestion, metabolism, elimination, body tone and strength, and bone density, and helps us normalize weight. When you choose the right exercise for you, it's enjoyable, increases self-worth, and brings you more energy. It can literally turn on our "smart genes," reverse aging, support emotional stability, and stave off depression.

The following benefits of exercise have long been proven scientifically.[21] Note that many if not all of these exercise-induced rewards directly correlate with risk for depression. Controlling blood sugar through exercise, for example, helps prevent blood sugar imbalances that masquerade as depression. And of course there's the lowered inflammation that's one of the most powerful ways in which exercise prevents depression. I'll get into the gist of that shortly, but for now take a look at all these marvelous benefits that go far beyond the mere physical:

▶ Increased stamina, strength, flexibility, and coordination
▶ Increased muscle tone and bone health
▶ Increased blood and lymph circulation and oxygen supply to cells and tissues
▶ More restful, sound sleep
▶ Balanced hormones
▶ Stress reduction and mood stability
▶ Increased self-esteem and sense of well-being
▶ Release of endorphins (brain chemicals) that act as natural mood lifters and pain relievers
▶ Decreased food cravings
▶ Decreased blood sugar levels and risk for diabetes
▶ Ideal weight distribution and maintenance
▶ Increased brain health, sharper memory, and lower risk for dementia
▶ Increased heart health and lower risk for cardiovascular disease
▶ Decreased inflammation and risk for age-related disease, including cancer
▶ Increased energy and productivity

Throughout most of our time on Earth, we've been physically active. But today modern technology has afforded us the privilege of a mostly sedentary existence. Science has even proven that over millions of years our genome evolved in a state of constant physical challenge—it took a massive amount of physical effort to find enough food just to survive. So our genome *expects* and *requires* frequent exercise.

Biologists Daniel E. Lieberman of Harvard and Dennis M. Bramble of the University of Utah know about the power of movement. Their research into the evolution of *Homo sapiens* and the penchant for running culminated in a highly referenced paper for the journal *Nature* in 2004 in which they assert that we've survived this long on the planet by virtue of our athleticism.[22] Our continual existence was fostered by our ancestors outrunning predators and hunting down valuable prey for food. We were able to find food and energy for mating, allowing the more active humans to pass on their genes to the next generation of stronger, hardier humans.

So what exactly is the science behind why exercise may be the panacea for the modern-day inflammation epidemic? There are multiple events that occur during exercise that bring about a reduction in inflammation. I'd like to highlight one recently discovered pathway that relates directly to depression. Although scientists have known that exercise seems to act as a buffer against depression, we haven't understood *how* exercise can lessen the risk for depression.[23] That is, until now, thanks to some clever new research conducted at the Karolinska Institute in Stockholm, Sweden, that examined the brains and behavior of mice.[24] Although we can't ask a mouse how they are feeling and if they are depressed, scientists have long been able to create parameters for knowing when a mouse is down and out based on behaviors that indicate depression in mice. These behaviors include declining tasty food, losing weight, and giving up trying to escape from an unpleasant environment (usually the cold-water maze). In this particular experiment, the researchers subjected mice to five weeks of low-level stress until the mice showed signs of depression. This was to be expected. But what would happen if the mice had run first—before being placed under stressful circumstances?

That's when the research got interesting. The scientists bred pre-exercised mice—a group of mice they forced to get fit before sending them on a proven path to depression. Previous research had already established that aerobic exercise in both mice and humans enhances the production of an enzyme called PGC-1alpha within muscles. Specifically, exercise increases levels of what's technically called PGC-1alpha1, a subtype of the enzyme. The Karolinska scientists theorized that this special enzyme protects the brain against depression by fostering certain conditions within the body. So to test their hypothesis, they created mice with high levels of PGC-1alpha1 even in the absence of exercise, as this allowed them to isolate the PGC-1alpha1 from other substances released by the muscles during and after exercise. Then the scientists exposed the rodents to five weeks of mild stress. And despite the stress, the mice didn't develop full-blown depression. When the researchers tried to figure out how this was happening, knowing that PGC-1alpha1 changes gene signaling, they turned to a substance called kynurenine, which accumulates in the bloodstream after stress and can even cross the blood-brain barrier. Kynurenine has been linked to depression because it's been shown to increase inflammation in the brain. In the mice with high levels of PGC-1alpha1, however, the kynurenine produced by stress was broken down by another protein expressed in response to signals from the PGC-1alpha1. And these broken-down parts could not pass the blood-brain barrier.

Did you catch that? That means that exercise can be a biological insurance plan against the bodily effects of stress.

The researchers didn't end their explorations there. They wanted to be sure that such findings were relevant to humans too. So they recruited a group of people willing to complete three weeks of frequent endurance training. The training involved forty to fifty minutes of moderate jogging or cycling. By taking muscle biopsies before and after the program, the scientists documented that the people's muscle cells had much more PGC-1alpha1 and the substance that breaks down kynurenine at the end of the program than at its start. The ultimate takeaway from these results in the simplest terms is that exercise lowers your risk of becoming depressed. Period.

Does the same biochemical processes likewise combat depression that already exists? That is yet to be determined. But this is promising news. Perhaps the process can be just as effective in treating depression as it is in preventing it. I know that my patients, even those who are the most depressed, feel the psychological rewards of exercise. Even my pregnant patients who engage in more movement find relief (and healthier, more enjoyable pregnancies). Now that may only sound like anecdotal evidence, but in the future the science will speak to this wisdom.

An entire book can be written about all the ways in which exercise boosts the body's physiology and, in turn, psychology. Bear in mind that multiple biological events take place in the body when we dance, take a cycling class, or go for a brisk walk. Exercise doesn't just positively change the body's physical chemistry, but can affect powerfully beneficial changes within the cells of our body down to the molecular and genetic levels. For instance, we now know that exercise directly affects the health of the mitochondria, which are your body's most important energy-producing structures. We have compelling proof of this from studies done on older folks who are placed on an exercise program and then compared with younger counterparts in terms of not only their strength and fitness levels but genetic changes. In one landmark 2007 experiment, for example, researchers studied the effects of six months of strength training in elderly volunteers aged sixty-five and older and discovered that exercise can partially help reverse the aging process.[25] Like the Karolinska researchers, they also took small biopsies of muscle cells from the participants before and after the program, then compared them with muscle cells from twenty-six young volunteers with an average age of twenty-two. The scientists, a team comprised of both Canadian and American researchers, recorded improved strength as well as significant changes at the genetic level that de-aged the older individuals.

Upon closer observation, the researchers realized that the genes that changed were involved in the functioning of mitochondria. More recent research has confirmed such findings, showing how high-intensity interval training positively stimulates mitochondrial biogenesis—essentially stimulating the regenerative process in these cells, resulting in the creation of more mitochondria.[26] Significant gains have been measured in as little as two weeks of interval training, which entails repeated bursts of high-energy output: you go hard for a short period, then ease up for a few minutes before resuming a higher level of intensity for another round.[27] This may in fact be better for you—and your mitochondria—than the long, slow and steady approach to exercise.

The health of your mitochondria is paramount to your general health, for their age and ability to perform have a direct correlation with your metabolic health, which in turn factors into your mental health. Your mitochondria are exceptionally vulnerable to cellular damage, which can result from a number of factors both under your control and not. In addition to your eating habits and environmental exposures, the amount of exercise you get also plays a vital role in your mitochondria's functionality and health, especially in determining how many mitochondria each cell type within your body has at its disposal (heart muscle, for instance, can have higher levels than skeletal muscle because it works tirelessly). Studies show that aerobic exercise for just fifteen to twenty minutes at a moderate intensity three to four times a week can increase the number of mitochondria in your muscle cells by a staggering 40 to 50 percent.[28] That's quite an exchange: a little bit of exercise for a huge increase in the amount of these little engines that rev up your energy metabolism.

Suffice it to say I'm going to ask you to start an exercise program if you don't already follow one. And I promise to make this doable even for the most exercise averse. You'll begin with five to ten minutes of burst exercise (thirty seconds of maximal effort and ninety seconds of recovery) and work up to twenty minutes three or more times a week. I'll give you plenty of ideas so you're sure to find something that you like.

CHAPTER 8

Clean House

How to Detoxify Your Environment

When in doubt, take it out.

Sadly, mainstream opinion upholds an "innocent until proven guilty" perspective when it comes to identifying and eliminating harmful chemicals, including drugs and environmental toxicants. We have seen this play out over time, from DDT to lead paint to cigarette smoking, and the more modern example, glyphosate. As scientists, we can't conduct traditional experiments to determine whether or not and how these chemicals affect people. It wouldn't be ethical to test certain exposures on a population to see what happens, and accounting for individual risk factors and timing of exposures is challenging.

So instead, we often resort to analyzing data gathered from accidents that happen, such as one in 1973 in Michigan, when cattle were unintentionally fed grain contaminated with the flame-retardant PBB, an estrogen mimicker. As a result, the PBB wound up in the meat and milk products from these animals. The girls born to women who had consumed those products started menstruating a year earlier than their peers on average. Or learn from our mistakes, such as the disastrous effects of DDT. DDT, an organochlorine pesticide that earned Dr. Paul Müller the Nobel Prize for its discovery in 1948, seemed like the clean and easy solution to mosquitos and all of the deadly diseases they traffic. My father grew up in New Jersey in the 1950s and vividly recalls running behind the spray of the trucks in the street (after playing with mercury beads in the Dumpster!). The infamous ad campaign jingled, "DDT is good for me!" After hundreds of millions had been exposed to DDT by 1970, there was still no discernible proof of human harm.

In response to rising concern and Rachel Carson's 1962 *Silent Spring* missive, thirty separate studies failed to find a link to breast cancer. That is, until the right study was done. Conducted by epidemiologist Barbara Cohn, her study of 20,000 pregnant women and children collected from 1959 to 1976 looked at medical records forty years later.[1] Because this study, which was just published in 2015, accounted for the science of epigenetics, vulnerable windows of exposure, and the role of hormones in carcinogenesis, it was able to detect a fivefold increase in breast cancer in those exposed to DDT spraying before puberty. Their children were at increased risk of breast and testicular cancer as well. DDT was banned in 1972, but it remains widespread in the environment and continues to be used in Africa and Asia. DDT was among the first recognized endocrine disruptors, and multiple studies now associate exposure to the chemical with reduced fertility, genital birth defects, diabetes, and damage to developing brains in addition to cancer.

And we can look at what happened following the bombings of Hiroshima and Nagasaki. Women who were under twenty when the atomic bombs hit had much higher rates of cancer and mental disorders when they grew up than women who were older at the time of the bombings. Pregnant women gave birth to children with similar health challenges throughout their lives, including neuropsychological disorders.

Medicine is under the influence of powerful lobbies and corporate interests that sway regulatory agencies and policymakers in the assessment of safety. Most doctors are convinced that the burden of proof lies with the sick patients and citizens to demonstrate that environmental exposures are at the root of their problems or an important contributor. Modern medicine has very little willingness to acknowledge the complexity and true origin of chronic illnesses that are the result of environmental, pharmaceutical, and dietary exposures. These ailments cannot be resolved by simply suppressing and managing symptoms, but the default medical approach is to turn off the smoke alarm while letting the fire rage on. The average internist does not appreciate how your genes, their expression, your hormonal milieu, and individual thresholds for toxic effects of environmental chemicals play out.

Unfortunately, doctors rarely make recommendations outside of medication for fear that the science does not support their interventions. The tide seems to be turning, however, with an increasing acceptance for the role of environmental exposures in contributing to disease. In 2014, the American College of Obstetrics released a bulletin that cautioned women about the harmful effects of plastics and flame retardants.[2] This was an important step because the chemical industry and their lobbyists have been working hard to suppress these concerns, and government regulators have followed suit.

In Part 1, I connected the dots between the toxicants that we encounter daily and mental health, in particular those that wreak havoc on our hormones and are thus called endocrine disruptors (EDCs). Flame retardants, for example, used widely in furniture, electronics, appliances, vehicles, clothing, and building materials, are notorious EDCs.[3] Exposures during pregnancy alone have been shown to adversely affect hormone and brain development in offspring. In fact, research shows that worldwide concentrations in humans and wildlife have been doubling every two to five years, with the exception of Sweden, where flame retardants are banned. In one of the first studies to examine the relationship between flame retardants and obesity, researchers fed mice a high-fat, high-calorie diet (the authors didn't disclose what type of "fat" they used) and found that those exposed to flame retardants gained 30 percent more weight than controls.[4] This has led to the labeling of these chemicals as obesogens, in that they accelerate weight gain, raise blood sugar, and contribute to metabolic disorders.[5]

Other common noxious chemicals, some of which I've mentioned earlier, include phthalates, perfluorinated chemicals, bisphenol A, arsenic, tributyltin, and chlorinated compounds such as dioxins, PCBs and DDT. Dioxins, for example, are a class of chemicals that are not only notorious for causing reproductive and developmental problems, damaging the immune system, and interfering with hormones, but are much easier to come into contact with than most people realize. Dioxins from chemical manufacturing with chlorine are mostly consumed through processed, nonorganic meat and dairy, and can even be released from seemingly innocuous, "natural" sweeteners like Splenda (sucralose) when heated, or leached from tampons.[6]

Now that you've learned how to minimize food sources of harmful chemicals, it's time to turn your attention to nondietary items such as household goods and products, cleaning supplies, plastic, clothing, water sources, cosmetics, toiletries and personal hygiene products, food and water storage, and invisible forms of pollution such as magnetic fields and questionable air quality.

I'll offer additional advice for women who are planning to become pregnant, are currently pregnant, or who are breast-feeding. Women in this stage of life need to be empowered to make the right decisions to protect themselves and their children. Indeed, the future of your child's mental wellness is directly impacted by exposures in utero. And I will admit that as one of the only physicians in the country with perinatal psychiatric training who takes a holistic, evidence-based approach, I can come across as a very protective mother bear in this department.

THE BODY BURDEN[7]

If you're a member of an industrialized nation, then you now have an average of seven hundred synthetic chemicals in your body from food, water, and air. The vast majority of these chemicals have not been thoroughly tested for potential health effects, or proved to be safe.

It seems like every other day we hear about an association between a chemical or contaminant in our environment and a health condition. And these toxicants are ubiquitous and difficult to avoid. In the past three decades, more than 100,000 chemicals have been approved for commercial use in the United States. Among these are more than 85,000 industrial chemicals, 10,000 food additives, 12,500 personal-care ingredients, 1,000 pesticide active ingredients, and scores of pharmaceutical drugs. Ever since the 1976 Toxic Substances Control Act (TSCA) was enacted, the Environmental Protection Agency (EPA) has required safety testing on only a small fraction of the chemicals listed on the TSCA chemical inventory. More than 8,000 of these substances are produced at annual volumes of 25,000 pounds or greater, and a ridiculously small percentage of them are regulated for safety by the EPA or the Food and Drug Administration.[8]

Those who keep up with the goings on in the world have become a lot more aware of chemicals in our environment in relation to climate change. The two go hand in hand in a lot of ways, as so many of the chemicals in use—whether industrial, agricultural, or food additives—contribute to the ecological damage underpinning these new climate patterns (more acidic oceans, for instance, or herbicides that irrevocably undermine soil health). Scientists have been measuring industrial pollutants in our environment for decades, but only recently have they begun the process of tracking the so-called body burden, the levels of toxicants in tissues of the human body. This biomonitoring, for which blood, urine, umbilical cord blood, and breast milk are analyzed, is being conducted by several high-profile institutions and research organizations worldwide. This includes top scientists working in either public, nationally funded organizations or private groups that analyze human tissues for industrial chemicals found in foods, air, water, and consumer products. The research of the various projects typically involves people of all ages (newborns to the elderly) from across the country. And these biomonitoring projects show that all US residents, no matter where they live or how old they are, contain measurable levels of synthetic chemicals. Most of these chemicals are fat-soluble and therefore stored in fatty tissue, where they biopersist (i.e., become parked). I care less about the monitoring and more about the actual policing of these chemicals. There is sufficient signal of harm to halt the production of certain chemicals such as Monsanto's Roundup, for example. Regulation and transparent oversight that controls for imbedded conflicts of interest will be our only way out of this chemical soup.

There's no single test you can take to determine your body burden and what that means for you in terms of risk for disease and depression. Testing for toxicants in the body isn't as easy as you might think. First, you'd have to know what to look for exactly, and second, you'd need a way to assess the effects that a given exposure is having on a given body. The fact that many toxicants hide deep in our tissues suggests that we as scientists have got much more to learn about our body's self-help mechanisms and the threshold at which they become overwhelmed.

Because studies report averages according to sex, age, and race, they cannot predict the body burdens of *individuals,* nor can they take into account all the possible contaminants or the potential for synergy between hundreds if not thousands of chemicals we are exposed to on a daily basis. Due to the fact that everyone's body reacts differently to external stimuli, including the effects of combinations of various stimuli, regulatory standards for limiting certain exposures to known pollutants may not protect uniquely vulnerable populations, such as women of reproductive age or people of any age with chronic illnesses or underlying genetic issues and susceptibilities.

UC Berkeley's Brenda Eskenazi is an epidemiologist and chief investigator of a notable study looking into the effects of very small amounts of pesticides on young children's brains. She's followed hundreds of pregnant women living in Salinas Valley, California, an agricultural center of gravity that has had up to a half million pounds of organophosphates sprayed in the region per year. In an article published in *The Nation,* she articulates the problem well:

"Throughout the course of a day, people may eat several different types of produce, each of which may bear traces of one or more pesticides. They encounter other types of chemicals as well—from antibacterials in soaps, to plasticizers in foodware, to flame retardants in the furniture. By day's end, you've got a combination of chemicals and an unknown level of risk."[9]

A synergy refers to chemical interactions between two substances. In isolation the substances can be relatively safe, but they can become harmful to us when combined. So a substance that's a 1 on a hypothetical danger scale of 1 to 10, and another that's a 4 can become a hazardous 8 when they encounter each other and react. Such a phenomenon, what some have also called the cocktail effect, ultimately means that the number of potential chemical toxicities is infinite.[10] As Randall Fitzgerald notes in his book *The Hundred Year Lie*, "What distresses and perplexes me is the realization that even if government had the resources to thoroughly conduct widespread safety testing—which it doesn't—our technology is too primitive to detect all of the synthetic chemicals in combination or to complete the task within our own lifetimes or even within the life spans of any of our grandchildren."[11] In September 2015, French researchers reported in a specialty journal for the prestigious *Nature* that some estrogens such as ethinylo estradiol (one of the active ingredients of contraceptive pills) and organochlorine pesticides, although very weakly active on their own, have the ability to bind simultaneously to a receptor located in the cell nucleus and to activate it synergistically.[12] Analyses at the molecular level indicate that the two compounds bind cooperatively to the receptor (meaning that binding of the first molecule promotes binding of the second). And the resulting mixture induces a toxic effect at substantially lower concentrations than the individual molecules.

Our body burden begins in utero and can last a lifetime. Although we used to think that the placenta acts as a shield, protecting cord blood from most chemicals and pollutants in the environment, we know differently now. Industrial chemicals and pollutants can indeed stream through the placenta just like residues from cigarettes and alcohol. Benchmark studies spearheaded by the nonprofit Environmental Working Group (EWG) first demonstrated this when they found chemicals in cord blood and breast milk, and other cutting-edge studies also have proven that wombs are not as bullet-proof as previously thought. Even the famous blood-brain barrier can be penetrated, especially in a developing fetus where it's not fully in place yet.

GET REAL AND REALISTIC

If you think you can move to a far-away land to find purity, think again. The by-products and chemicals from industrial centers have landed in our world's (previously) most pristine areas through air and water currents. In the air, dust particles glom on to chemicals and travel north to colder climates. This helps explain why animals and humans who live thousands of miles from sources of pollution show signs of contamination. And the same is true in waters that are thousands of miles away from industrial areas. Jet streams and water currents can make two remote places practically neighbors. Whales are high enough on the food chain that some bioaccumulate enough PCBs in their fatty tissues to render their carcasses as hazardous waste in some cases. Inuit women who inhabit the Arctic regions have been shown to have PCBs in their breast milk. These exposures have been shown to affect the health of their children.

We would like to assume our elected representatives will protect us by not allowing harmful chemicals to be used or sold in this country, but that assumption would be false. Instead, Congress has limited or cut the EPA's budget for the past decade. One reason for this is pure politics: some members of Congress place a higher priority on protecting the interests of industry and business than on public health. And the regulations imposed by state and local governments are highly variable in the degree of attention given to environmental health.

Budgetary constraints and giving in to powerful lobbies also stymie the effectiveness of the very federal agencies that are supposed to protect us: the FDA, which enforces the regulations on the levels of chemicals, pesticides, and other additives permitted in foods and drugs; the USDA, which regulates agricultural use of pesticides (along with the EPA), hormones, and antibiotics; and the Department of Labor, which enforces the Occupational Safety and Health Act of 1970 to address exposure to toxic substances in the workplace.

Bottom line: it's impossible to know how many synthetic chemicals exist in the world today and how harmful they really are, especially in combination. It's also impossible to rely on laws or regulations to protect you, given the competing myriad political interests.

ONE THING AT A TIME[13]

I wasn't always a clean living crusader. But pregnancy has a way of turning on that just-tell-me-what-to-do-to-get-this-right-NOW switch. Several years ago, that switch was activated for me when a friend gave me *Green Babies, Sage Moms* when I was expecting my first baby. As I read that book, I realized that doctors aren't taught to help women optimize health and wellness. It was up to me to learn how to clean up my home and my body, one step at a time.

I can still visualize my garbage can after this epiphany—it overflowed with bathroom products that had been instantly rendered biohazards of the first degree. Even Kiehl's? I shook my head in amazement at the seductive power of the word *natural* in advertising. Ever since my realization, I have been on a mission to disseminate information that will help women vote with their wallets for the betterment of their health and their babies. It's crucial for us to know what steps we can take.

For those who worry that what they do might not make a

difference in the face of these persistent environmental hazards, I tell them that it is like stepping outside into a freezing blizzard: if you only put on a couple layers of clothes, it's still a whole lot better than braving the elements fully naked!

While it may seem like an overwhelming task to clear out your house of questionable products and replace them with alternatives, it needn't be stressful. Go one room or one product at a time; I'll be helping you do that during week 2 of the program (see Chapter 10). The goal is to do the best you can based on what you can afford and what you're willing to change. Keep it simple by buying products that are as close to their natural state as possible—ones that haven't been processed, treated, grown, manufactured, or infused with chemicals in any way.

Use the EWG's user-friendly website (www.ewg.org), Fearless Parent (www.fearlessparent.org), I Read Labels For You (www.ireadlabelsforyou.com), and Healthy Home Economist (www.thehealthyhomeeconomist.com) to search for the safest products and lifestyle tips. Remember, it can take more than a decade for studies to gather enough evidence before new standards or regulations pass, or dangerous products are taken off the market. A meta-analysis published in the *Journal of Hazardous Materials* in 2014 reviewed 143,000 peer-reviewed papers to track the patterns of emergence and decline of toxic chemicals.[14] Shockingly, this study revealed that fourteen years is an average time span between the onset of initial safety concerns and the height of concern and appropriate action. Emblematic of this pattern are DDT, perchlorate, 1,4-dioxane, triclosan, nanomaterials, and microplastics making their way into the environment and our homes. Such a finding echoes the seventeen-year lag in scientific data making its way into the doctor's office. What this suggests is that we need to take matters into our own hands.

The best you can do today is use common sense and sound judgment based on current science. Put simply: don't wait until a product or ingredient is officially labeled "dangerous" to remove or extremely limit it from your life; when in doubt, take it out of your life. Below is a guide to performing an easy cleanup.

In the Kitchen

▶ Avoid canned foods, which you should be doing anyhow if you follow my dietary protocol, and stick with fresh, whole foods. Cans are often lined with a BPA-laden coating.

▶ Don't use nonstick pans or cookware. Teflon-coated wares contain perfluorooctanoic acid, or PFOA, which even the EPA has labeled a likely carcinogen. Cast-iron, ceramic, or glass cookware are your best bet. Look online for used pans and pots made of these materials.

▶ Ditch the microwave and never put hot foods in plastic, which can release nasty chemicals that are absorbed by the food.

▶ Stop using plastic water bottles (or at least avoid plastics marked with a *PC,* for polycarbonate, or the recycling labels 3, 6, and 7 on the little triangle). Buy reusable bottles made of food-grade stainless steel or glass. Good old-fashioned glass is the most inert container to cook with and store hot foods in. You can buy a set of glass containers for less than $40 and be assured of a long life span.

In the Bathroom

▶ When it comes to toiletries, deodorants, soaps, cosmetics, and general beauty products, remember that our skin is a major entry point to our bodies, and what we slather on our skin and lips may make its way to our more vulnerable parts. Look for the genuine USDA organic seal and choose products that are safer alternatives (go to www.ewg.org for lists and re-sources). Find phthalate-free personal care products by using the Environmental Working Group's Skin Deep Cosmetics Database, www.ewg.org/skindeep and be wary of vinyl shower curtains.

Avoid the following ingredients, many of which are potential EDCs:

Triclosan and triclocarban (antibacterial hand soaps and some toothpastes)

Formaldehyde and formalin (nail products)

Toluene and dibutyl phthalate (DBP; nail polish)

TEA (triethanolamine)

"Fragrance" and "parfum"

Parabens (methyl-, propyl-, isopropyl-, butyl-, and isobutyl-)

PEG/ceteareth/polyethylene glycol

Diethyl phthalate

Sodium lauryl sulfate (SLS), sodium laureth sulfate (SLES), and ammonium lauryl sulfate (ALS)

Aluminum chlorohydrate (deodorants)

Sephora has a growing line of green cosmetics and grocers such as Whole Foods are a good place to start, although you'll still need to scan labels for any of the above agents of concern. For sunscreen, I use ones that contain non-micronized zinc and are free of oxybenzone such as Badger brand. Natural bug sprays like Bite Blocker and California Baby use alternatives to harmful DEET such as essential oils.

I recommend that you keep a skin brush in the bathroom for dry skin brushing (body brushing), a method of stimulating and cleansing the lymphatic system and detoxifying the skin. Remember, lymph flow is directly related to your immune and detoxification systems. However simple it may seem, it is a very powerful, effective technique. Use a brush with soft natural vegetable bristles or a loofah sponge, which you can find in most natural food stores and department stores. Keep the brush or sponge dry and pass it over your dry skin in a clean sweeping motion—no back-and-forth or scrubbing motions and move it in the direction of the lower abdomen—up the legs, up the arms, and down the neck and trunk, everywhere but your face. Do this twice a day, or up to four times a day during times of intense toxicity.

Go organic "down there": trash your tampons
In 2013, the "Chem Fatale" report by the Women's Voices for the Earth organization explored the loopholes that allow for toxic chemicals in feminine products to go untested and unpoliced.[15] For those of you who love your monthly supply, you're not going to want to hear this: most commercial tampons and pads contain dioxins, furans, and pesticides associated with cancer and endocrine/reproductive disruption.[16] Wipes, washes, douches, and deodorants contain parabens, dyes, and unknown chemicals under the label of "fragrance." These products are in intimate contact with mucosal tissue in girls, now beginning at precocious ages, and up through menopause.

We cannot rely on the FDA to assure the safety of these products, classified as "medical devices" (tampons) and "cosmetics" (such as wipes). Choose an inert method such as GladRags or organic feminine products.

Ditch hand sanitizers
The study's title says it all: "Holding Thermal Receipt Paper and Eating Food after Using Hand Sanitizer Results in High Serum Bioactive and Urine Total Levels of Bisphenol A (BPA)." Yikes. This is what a consortium from the University of Missouri discovered in 2014, publishing their findings in the *Public Library of Science* journal.[17] Turns out that those ubiquitous hand sanitizers, as well as other commercial skin care products, contain potent mixtures of chemicals that enhance the penetration of substances through the skin—by up to two hundred–fold. Most of these hand sanitizers, many of which are alcohol based, have been proven to be ineffective and likely kill the beneficial bacteria that are our most potent ally. So I encourage you to avoid these products entirely, but if you must, use an essential oil–based product that's all-natural.

Wash your hands the old-fashioned way with soap and water. And decline those cashier receipts that contain toxic substances like bisphenol A (BPA) and its equally toxic cousin bisphenol S (BPS) in an amount as high as 3 percent by weight.

General Household Goods

▶ Ventilate your home well and install HEPA air filters if possible. Change your air-conditioning and heating filters every three to six months and get the ducts cleaned yearly. Avoid air deodorizers and plug-in room fresheners. Indoor air is notoriously more toxic than outdoor air due to all the particulate matter that comes from furniture, electronics, and household goods. Request that people take off their shoes when they enter your house.

▶ Reduce toxic dust and residues that you cannot see or smell from furniture, electronics, and textiles by using a vacuum cleaner with a HEPA filter.

▶ Keep as many plants in your home as possible, as they naturally detoxify the environment. Spider plants, aloe vera, chrysanthemums, Gerbera daisies, Boston ferns, English ivies, and philodendrons are good choices. Use fifteen to twenty plants per 1,800 square feet.

▶ Be cautious about toys made before 2009, as they may contain dangerous plastics and treated materials. Avoid anything with that "new plastic" smell, such as beach inflatables.

▶ Until you can purchase an organic mattress, buy 100 percent all-natural covers that fit snugly to prevent "off-gassing" chemicals from passing through the sheets. And use hypoallergenic pillows filled with natural fibers such as cotton, wool, or feathers.

▶ The next time you're in the market for a new couch or bed, choose one made without toxic adhesives and glues (such as those containing formaldehyde), toxic plastics, synthetic wood or particleboard, and treated wood.

▶ When purchasing clothes, fabrics, upholstered furniture, or mattresses, choose ones that are free of flame-retardant, stain-resistant, and water-resistant coatings. Avoid reupholstering foam furniture.

▶ Hire an expert to replace old carpet; the padding may contain polybrominated diphenyl ethers (PBDEs). When refurbishing your home, start with flooring, because carpets in particular are magnets for dust and toxic chemicals. Go for natural hard-wood, cork, or carpets made with all-natural fibers that haven't been treated with flame-retardant or stain-resistant chemicals. Synthetic carpets can "off-gas" chemicals for years, which can affect the health of sensitive people.

▸ Whenever you buy household cleaners, detergents, disinfectants, bleach, stain removers, and so on, select ones that are free of synthetic chemicals (basically anything that looks suspicious in the list of ingredients). Most commercial cleaning products have a dauntingly long list of ingredients, and learning which ingredients to avoid can seemingly require a chemistry degree. Ammonia-containing glass cleaners and bleach, for example, emit toxins into our homes. Do not depend on labels that say "safe," "nontoxic," "green," or "natural," because these terms have no legal meaning. Read labels carefully and pay special attention to warnings. Don't buy any products labeled "poison," "danger," or "fatal" if swallowed or inhaled. Avoid anything with the following ingredients: diethylene glycol monoethyl ether, 2-butoxyethanol (EGBE), and methoxydiglycol (DEGME). Stick with trusted brands that feature minimal ingredients on the label (see my website for brand recommendations). Or make your own: simple, inexpensive, and effective cleaning products can be made from borax, baking soda, and water for a scrubbing paste; vinegar and water for wipe downs; and lemon. The simplest all-purpose cleaner consists of 1 teaspoon vinegar in 2 cups water. Throw in some essential oils like a drop or two of peppermint if you want to get fancy! For more details and product information, go to www.ewg.org and www.fearlessparent.org.

▸ Wet mop floors and wipe down windowsills weekly.

▸ Speak with your local garden store or nursery personnel for recommendations on pesticide- and herbicide-free products to control pests. And don't use leaded pottery (hardware stores have inexpensive, easy-to-use kits to determine whether your favorite flower bowl has lead in it).

About Your Faucets

Municipal water is contaminated with pharmaceutical products, industrial pollutants, microbes, and about six hundred different toxic-disinfecting by-products.[18] Additionally, it is processed with endocrine-disrupting and neurotoxic fluoride and chlorine. The Environmental Working Group has identified 316 water contaminants, 202 of which are not regulated (or understood). And don't think that you're "safe" because you live in a good neighborhood. In 2013, a study led by Princeton University in collaboration with researchers from Columbia University and the University of California, San Diego, found that pregnant women living in areas with contaminated drinking water may be more likely to have babies that are premature or with low birth weights (considered less than 5.5 pounds).[19]

This particular study examined ten years of New Jersey birth records and data on drinking-water quality collected from 1997 to 2007. They uncovered violation records across 488 water districts in New Jersey, finding that more than a quarter of them had water contamination violations that affected more than 30,000 people.[20] The violations included both chemical and bacterial contamination, such as dichloroethane, a solvent often used for plastics or as a degreaser, as well as radon and coliform. When a water district is affected, the Department of Environmental Protection is required to send all residences notices, but these notices often go, well, unnoticed and discarded as junk mail.

I urge you to buy a household water filter for all of your drinking and cooking purposes. There are a variety of water treatment technologies available today, from simple filtration pitchers you fill manually to under-the-sink contraptions or units designed to filter the water coming into your home from its source. I'm a big fan of the systems that employ reverse osmosis and carbon filters; check those out if possible. It's up to you to decide which one best suits your circumstances and budget. Make sure the filter you buy removes fluoride, chlorine, and other potential contaminants.

Many of these filters, even below-the-sink models, can move with you when you leave.

It's important that whichever filter you choose, you maintain it well and follow the manufacturer's directions to make sure it continues to perform. As contaminants build up, a filter will become less effective, and it can then start to release chemicals back into your filtered water. You might also think about putting filters on your showerheads. Shower filtration systems are easy to find and inexpensive and eliminate your exposure to vaporized chlorine and its natural carcinogenic by-product chloroform.

Ring Ring: About That Cell Phone

Cellular phones have become an indispensable tool for many of us in the modern world. But they can be evil in ways that go beyond just keeping us plugged in all the time and feeling like we need to respond to incoming messages and texts as soon as possible. The jury is no longer still out pondering the physical consequences to having these electronics hugging our ears: new data shows that your cell phone is not only a carcinogenic, radiation-emitting device, but it may alter the structure and function of your brain, including brain wave activity that is intimately connected to cognition, mood, and behavior.

In 2015, a disconcerting new clinical study emerged from researchers in the Netherlands and King's College revealing that so-called third-generation (3G) cell phone technology induces widespread brain wave activity in people in as little as fifteen minutes of "talk time" with the phone held up to the ear area.[21]

First our bodies use very delicate electrical impulses to exist. Our brains send messages to the muscles, glands, and so on not only using chemicals but also using electrical currents that, for example, are measured with an electroencephalogram. The workings inside each one of our cells are controlled by very small electrical impulses.

This wasn't the first time that researchers have addressed the question of whether cell phones can be hazardous. Earlier research found that they can affect alpha brain wave activity, and subsequent behavioral challenges, notably insomnia.[22] But this was the first placebo-controlled, single-blind study of its kind to show that modern cell phone technology can, within minutes, be "associated with increased activity of the alpha, beta, and gamma frequency bands in nearly every brain region." In other words, typical cell phone exposure resulted in electrophysiological changes big enough to measure in nearly the entire brain's structure and function. We all know that cell phone radiation can disrupt certain equipment, which is why you have to use "airplane mode" on a plane, but we seem to disregard the fact that it may adversely affect our brains, which is an electrical impulse sensitive organ.

It helps to remember that our bodies use very delicate electrical impulses to exist. Our brains send messages to the muscles and glands not only using chemicals but electrical currents as well. And the workings inside each one of our cells are controlled by very small electrical impulses. Children are more likely to be vulnerable to the type of radiation produced by tablets, mobile phones, and Wi-Fi. In several countries in Europe, Wi-Fi has been banned in schools.

Why has it taken us so long to know about potentially mind-altering properties of cell phone radiation? The electrical-based technologies developed over the last sixty years may be interfering with the inner workings of our bodies in ways we just can't quantify yet. Many brain cancers, for example, are only visible after many years of frequent mobile phone use.

Almost most of the studies on cell phone exposure have turned up inconclusive findings on cognition, as much as 87 percent of brain wave studies looking at the effects of cellular electromagnetic radiation are funded by the mobile phone industry.[23] Since 2011, cell phone radiation has been classified by the International Agency for Research on Cancer as "possibly carcinogenic." And because brain waves are believed to encode our behavior, it's reasonable to assume that altering their activity could have downstream effects on behavior and consciousness—even if the concerns raised don't seem to warrant reduced usage.

Don't panic: I won't ask you to ditch your cell phone. If anyone knows how unrealistic that is, it's me. You can certainly reduce your exposure by not putting the phone up against your head (use an air tube headset), keeping it more than six feet from your body when possible. And remember that you can put your phone on airplane mode if you or your child is handling it without the need for cellular Wi-Fi. Simple precautions like these can greatly reduce you and your loved ones' risk of adverse health effects associated with exposure.

Magnetic fields, an invisible form of pollution that's totally understudied, should be minimized. For this reason I recommend that you budget in extra time at the airport to request a pat-down instead of going through the full body scanner and subjecting your DNA to ionizing radiation in advance of the inevitable radiation from the flight.

A NOTE TO PREGNANT WOMEN AND NEW MOTHERS

I treat all my patients like pregnant women because if it's not safe for a baby, why would it be totally fine for an adult? That said, I should reiterate that the cautionary and instructional notes in this chapter couldn't be more pertinent to women who are planning to become pregnant, who are pregnant now, or who are breastfeeding. From choosing natural products to drinking pure water free of chemicals, doing what you can to protect the health of your baby is paramount in your role as a mother. It will go a long way to preserve your health and mental wellness as well as that of your child.

If you're expecting, you should know that if for whatever reason you undergo a C-section, researchers are deep in the process of trying to help replace what's lost by going through that procedure. Dr. Maria Gloria Dominguez-Bello of New York University's Human Microbiome Project has presented research suggesting that

using gauze to collect a mother's birth-canal bacteria and then im-
parting them to a baby born by C-section by rubbing the gauze
over their mouths and noses helps make those babies' bacterial populations more closely resemble vaginally born babies.[24] It's not a
substitute for having a vaginal delivery, but it's better than a ster-
ile C-section. This, along with the strategies I've outlined in this
chapter, will equip your baby with a metaphorical bulletproof vest
against the assaults he or she will encounter.

CHAPTER 9

Testing and Supplementing

Supporting the Healing Process

The twelve simple, noninvasive lab tests your doctor isn't ordering.

Consider the following scenario, something typical of what I witness in my office: a lovely thirty-something woman comes in to see me. She says she has a debilitating and highly agitated form of depression, no energy, and brain fog. I even note some instability when she walks. When I take her history, she tells me she was put on an acid-blocking medication two years ago for her heartburn. I ask about her diet, which is high in sugar, gluten, dairy, and "convenient" fried foods, all of which are likely the root of her reflux. It's well known clinically and in the research literature that long-term suppression of stomach acid blocks the absorption of the essential B_{12} vitamin.[1]

Vitamin B_{12}, as you know by now, is one of the basic building blocks of life. And it's one of the all-star antidepressants. We all need vitamin B_{12} to make red blood cells and nerve cell lining and to regulate the expression of our DNA and multiple other brain and body-based functions. It protects the brain and nervous system, regulates rest and mood cycles, and keeps the immune system functioning properly. A severe deficiency can lead to deep depression, paranoia and delusions, memory loss, incontinence, and loss of taste and smell, among other serious conditions. The medical literature is filled with case reports of people with these conditions that a single shot of vitamin B_{12} cured. Babies born to a mother deficient in B_{12} are at serious risk for neurological symptoms such as lethargy, developmental delays, and delayed cognitive and motor development.[2]

A B_{12} deficiency has tremendous consequences. It cripples the ability of nerves to communicate and transmit messages, and it can lead to depression, confusion, and, eventually, physical brain shrinkage and dementia.[3] It's standard in my practice to order a simple blood test to determine B_{12} levels in patients. It's practically a no-brainer for me today, as I know I can meaningfully move the health needle for many patients with this simple intervention. B_{12} is replaced in the body with a prescribed injection or a nonprescription tablet that is dissolved under the tongue. Which might make you wonder: Are you deficient in just vitamin B_{12} or some other vital ingredient your body needs to thrive as well? Could you extinguish your depression through a supplement?

As a prelude to starting the thirty-day program, I'm going to outline two key features of my general protocol: testing and supplementing. In other words, ordering certain laboratory tests to determine your baseline and rule out underlying medical conditions and deficiencies and learning about which supplements and noninvasive therapies might also help you. While I won't ask you to start supplementing until after two weeks of lifestyle and diet change, it helps to know what kind of daily supplement regimen you may want to consider further down the road. The reason for this is that supplementation and its benefits will be most notable after the sometimes challenging transition to a whole foods diet. Let me add that I sit in a place of nonattachment to testing and supplementation because what we think we know today may shift or be outdated tomorrow. Even more dogmatic perspectives such as "vitamin D is good for everyone" and "folic acid is always bad" need to be held gently. So keep that in mind as you read through this chapter and begin to think of the ways in which you'll customize the program to your needs and unique circumstances.

I'll start by giving you a rundown of medical tests and laboratory studies you may want to order with your doctor. Most of these can be done as soon as you're ready to schedule an appointment and request these from your practitioner.

TESTING TESTING, 1-2-3

Below are the twelve tests I most commonly use with my patients. I've included target healthy levels where appropriate.

Thyroid Function Tests

While there are limitations to the ability of conventional blood tests to detect functional hypothyroidism, this panel demonstrates how well your thyroid gland is functioning, whether the brain is sensing hormone levels, what those levels are, and whether or not the immune system is mistakenly attacking the gland. As a recap, thyroid hormone production is controlled by a feedback loop among your thyroid gland, pituitary gland, and hypothalamus. Hypothalamic thyrotropin-releasing hormone (TRH) stimulates pituitary thyrotropin (TSH) synthesis and secretion. TSH then triggers production and release of T4 and T3 from the thyroid gland. When enough T4 is produced, it signals to TRH and TSH that there is plenty in circulation and to halt production. About 85 percent of the hormone produced by our thyroid gland is T4, which is a relatively inactive form of the hormone. A small amount of T4 gets converted into the active form of thyroid hormone, T3. This molecule also gets converted into either free T3 (FT3) or reverse T3 (RT3).

Free T3 is important, as it's the primary thyroid hormone that can attach to a receptor and have a direct effect on your physiology. T3 is one of the body's master molecules. It commands your metabolism and how your body uses energy, controls body temperature, maintains the movement of your bowels, and keeps other hormones in check. Although we don't know exactly what reverse T3 does, it tends to be elevated in people who are experiencing bodily stress as a means of slowing down and conserving energy for recovery. Most conventional doctors use only one or two tests (TSH and T4) to screen for problems. They don't check free T3 (FT3), reverse T3 (RT3), or thyroid antibodies. As I mentioned earlier, the autoimmune disease Hashimoto's thyroiditis is the most common form of hypothyroidism in women. I screen for it routinely in my patients by ordering thyroid peroxidase antibodies (TPOAb) and thyroglobulin antibodies (TgAb). Here's my roundup of thyroid tests that I implore you to have your doctor order. No one should be treating hypothyroidism with Zoloft, if you know what I mean. This will gauge your thyroid health (optimal values included):

TSH: optimal value: less than 2 μU/ML

FREE T4: optimal value: more than 1.1 NG/DL

FREE T3: optimal value: more than 3.0 PG/ML

REVERSE T3: optimal value: less than a 10:1 ratio RT3:FT3

THYROID PEROXIDASE ANTIBODIES (TPOAB): optimal value: less than 4 IU/ML or negative

THYROGLOBULIN ANTIBODIES (TGAB): optimal value: less than 4 IU/ML or negative

Already taking Synthroid or been told you should for your underperforming thyroid? If you have received the label of hypothyroidism, you'll remain obliquely objectified by your lab work as your doctors use synthetic T4—Synthroid—to attempt to move your TSH within range, more often leaving you symptomatic but "treated" because of poor conversion to active thyroid hormone (T3) and suppression of natural T3 production because of your now lower TSH. In this way, women are told that they are "fine," as my colleague Datis Kharrazian wrote in his book *Why Do I Still Have Thyroid Symptoms When My Lab Tests Are Normal?* If detected early, thyroid autoimmunity can be reversed and I am living proof. Even after years on synthetic replacement or after thyroid gland removal, patients can be returned to more optimal health with a natural form of thyroid hormone, what's called a desiccated thyroid replacement that contains all of the factors from animal thyroid tissue (usually coming from pigs). So if your doctor recommends a thyroid replacement drug, ask about alternatives to Synthroid and follow through the protocol in this book. Remember: optimization of lifestyle factors, especially via diet, remains a critical first intervention to resolve potential thyroid dysfunction.

MTHFR (Methylation)

The MTHFR gene produces the MTHFR enzyme (methylenetetrahydrofolate reductase), which is essential for several bodily processes that directly tie into mental well-being. When it's working right, the MTHFR gene begins a multistep chemical breakdown process called methylation, which ultimately helps you to make important proteins, use antioxidants, combat inflammation, eliminate toxins and heavy metals, keep homocysteine within normal range, optimize brain function, and silence the genes in your body (methylation) whose overexpression could cause harm. A defect in the MTFHR gene is highly correlated with psychiatric symptoms. There are two common variants to this gene wherein replacements of single nucleotides (pieces of DNA) results in lesser functioning. Every day we are learning more about the true clinical significance of variants to the 1298 and C677 gene locations. One mutation means your enzyme is functioning at 70 percent, and two defects can mean you're down to 30 percent. These mutations are not as rare as you might think. In the eight years I've been routinely testing for this gene in my patients, I've only had five patients who do *not* have a variation. So don't panic if you test positive for one or both inherited mutations. It just means that you need to be aware of your higher-than-normal risk for deficiencies as a result and for which supplementing activated folate (called methylfolate) and its partner, B_{12}, is likely indicated. (Note: the actual test for this defect is simply called the MTHFR mutation test.)

Vitamin B$_{12}$

The test that measures serum vitamin B$_{12}$ levels. Some two-fifths of the population are severely deficient in B$_{12}$ for a variety of reasons, from poor diet and dysbiosis (a disrupted gut flora) to use of medications like acid-reflux and diabetes drugs. Deficiency is traditionally defined as being below 150 to 200 pg/mL (picogram/milliliter), but you want to be above 600 pg/mL.

It turns out that testing for deficiency by blood level is not always a reliable indicator of what is going on in the brain or, functionally, in the body. Which is why it helps to look at levels of homocysteine and methylmalonic acid—two surrogate markers for levels of B$_{12}$, as well.

Homocysteine and methylmalonic acid

As I mentioned above, this is a more accurate and more sensitive method of screening for vitamin B$_{12}$ deficiency, especially when it's considered within the context of results from a basic red blood cell test. When these two substances are elevated in the blood, it's an indication that B$_{12}$ is low. Homocysteine is an inflammatory protein that must be metabolized by B$_{12}$ and folate, and methylmalonic acid is a compound that reacts with vitamin B$_{12}$ to produce coenzyme A, which is essential to normal cellular function. Optimal levels of homocysteine are between 7 and 10 micromoles per liter of blood; normal levels of methylmalonic acid are between 0.08 and 0.56 mmol/L (in my experience, this is a less sensitive measure). Typically a homocysteine over 8 is a red flag for inflammation that may be responsive to B$_{12}$ supplementation.

Hs-CRP (High-Sensitive C-Reactive Protein)

C-reactive protein is a protein the liver makes when there are general inflammatory messengers in the body. It can be measured with an hs-CRP test. You want to be between 0.00 and 1.0 mg/L.

Fasting Glucose/Insulin/HbA1C (Hemoglobin A1C)

The purpose of these tests is to check blood sugar control. The HgA1C test is the most accurate because it can give an average of your blood sugar levels over the past ninety days (the average life cycle of a red blood cell). You want your values to be between 4.8 and 5.2 percent (note anemia and dehydration can lead to falsely depressed or elevated levels). Fasting glucose is a onetime snapshot in the fasting state, of course, but should ideally be 70 to 85 mg/dl with a fasting insulin below 6 µIU/ml.

A glucose tolerance test also can assess for hypoglycemia, but clinically, reactive hypoglycemia is typically very obvious—these are the patients who wake up full but who can't go more than two hours without getting "hangry," shaky, or light-headed and feel progressively worse over the day.

Vitamin D

This test measures serum levels of this important hormone–vitamin. I test all of my patients for not just vitamin D (expressed clinically as 25OH), but also its receptor-activating metabolite (1,25). Ideally 25OH should be between 50 and 80 ng/mL; 1,25 should be within normal range. Don't be alarmed if your vitamin D level is abysmally low. There are reasons for low vitamin D beyond lack of sunlight, including the effects of widespread pesticide exposure on our liver's ability to produce vitamin D. The majority of Americans are deficient in this critical nutrient, and it can take time for the body to shore up its levels of vitamin D upon supplementation (see below).

Salivary Cortisol

The body has two adrenal glands, one located above each kidney. Hormones secreted by these endocrine glands help to regulate many body processes that impact mental health. Testing adrenal function through measuring levels of adrenal hormones in saliva and urine can be illuminating but in my experience is usually just visual confirmation of the known fact: we are under chronic, unremitting stress. A screening test of salivary cortisol measures levels of the stress hormone cortisol at four points in the day (usually at 8 a.m., noon, 4 p.m., and between 11 p.m. and midnight). Although it doesn't tell you about what the hormone is doing at the receptor, how it is being broken down, or what has caused cortisol production to change, the test is nevertheless useful to explain symptoms and their timing because the pattern of cortisol output changes throughout the day and should naturally be higher in the morning and lower at night.

All you'll have to do is spit into a test tube at those designated times and mail the tubes back to the lab for analysis (refrigeration is not necessary). This type of testing can also be extended to include sex hormones like progesterone and estrogen in the week before a woman's menstrual cycle, or even daily throughout the month. In fact, cortisol is not just your main adrenal hormone, it's made from progesterone, so every molecule of cortisol you produce when you're under stress depletes your progesterone levels. This explains why bouts of stress can cause premature hot flashes.

Note: these tests should be done *after* the thirty days of the program, particularly if sleep-related symptoms persist.

Stool PCR Testing

This type of test evaluates your gastrointestinal function and can detect imbalances in your gut microbiota, the presence of parasites, absorption issues, and gut inflammation. While we are still in the process of elucidating the "optimal" microbiome, important variables are levels of beneficial bacteria, any notable infections that may correlate with inflammatory markers in this test (just because a result shows a particular parasite, for example, does not necessarily mean that this is a problem for a given individual's ecology), and evidence of poor digestion. Since diet can change within days, this test is probably also best to do *after* the first thirty days on the program if you feel it's necessary.

Urinary Organic Acid Test

This test, which measures certain molecules found in urine, offers a view into the body's cellular metabolic processes. It can tell if there's a defect somewhere in your body's metabolism. I rarely need to perform this test and reserve it for cases of more complex fatigue and cognitive symptoms.

THE TEST CHECKLIST

The following list of tests should be ordered by your doctor:

Ideally before the thirty days to establish your baseline:

Thyroid function tests: TSH, free T4, free T3, reverse T3, thyroid peroxidase antibodies, and thyroglobulin antibodies	The MTHFR genetic test Vitamin B_{12} levels in blood Homocysteine levels in blood Hs-CRP	(high-sensitive C-reactive protein) in blood Fasting glucose/insulin/HbA1C (hemoglobin A1C) Vitamin D levels via 25OH and 1,25

After the thirty days, you can repeat the above tests and also consider:

Salivary cortisol	Stool culture, PCR, and proteomic testing	Urinary organic acid test

---

If your doctor won't order some of these tests, you may have to go elsewhere. The MTHFR gene test, for example, is not one routinely ordered by general internists. A naturopath or functional medicine doctor is more likely to know about this test and the current interpretation of its results. Be your own advocate and demand this baseline assessment; most of these tests are either covered by insurance or are relatively inexpensive. Proper diagnosis can go a long way in identifying the best support during the healing phase.

Upon completion of the four-week program, these laboratory studies should be repeated, though it may take several months of repeat testing to see dramatic improvement in these areas. C-reactive protein, for example, may take several months to improve. The same goes for hemoglobin A1C, which is typically measured in only three-to-four month intervals. But from day one of the program, you should begin to see positive changes in your blood glucose and insulin levels, and that will motivate you to keep going.

SUPPLEMENTS[4]

I wish we lived in a world where supplementation wasn't necessary. I wish we lived in a world in which detox was only a gimmick to sell spa treatments. Unless you are growing your own organic food in a bubble hermetically sealed from the ravages of the modern industrial world, strategic supplementation is almost always going to help you get better and stay better. My "menu" of supplements can get lengthy, so here I've broken my list down into two categories: the core basics and some additional considerations. I recommend that you consider all the core basics, and then add other supplements as you see fit given your unique circumstances. It is clearly preferable to work with a practitioner versed in the use of these supplements, and each should be started one at a time (with at least a day between a new supplement initiation) to observe for any immediate effect. Note that because supplements can help to support detoxification, they should be stopped in their entirety for five days every twenty days to allow the body to recalibrate.

Core Basics: B Vitamins, Minerals, Fatty Acids, Glandulars, and Digestive Enzymes

Activated B Complex
The B vitamins are the body's prime molecules for making mood-building biochemicals. They are thiamin (B_1), riboflavin (B_2), niacin

(B_3), pyridoxine (B_6), folate (B_9), vitamin B_{12}, biotin, and pantothenic acid (B_5). These vitamins help the body convert food into fuel and metabolize fats and protein. They are needed for healthy skin, hair, eyes, and liver and they help the adrenal glands and nervous system function properly. All eight B vitamins are water-soluble, so the body cannot store them. While gut bacteria help produce most of them, supplementing would help to ensure we meet our needs.

A large 2010 study led by researchers at Rush University looked at more than 3,500 adults and showed that higher intakes of B_6, B_9, and B_{12}—whether through foods or supplementation—was associated with a decreased likelihood of depression for up to twelve years of follow-up.[5] And for each additional 10 mg of vitamin B_6 and additional 10 μg of vitamin B_{12}, there was a 2 percent decreased risk of depressive symptoms per year.

The key to supplementing with a B complex vitamin is to get the best forms of the nutrients. Some forms may be less effective or even dangerous when taken in excess. Folate, for example, is the vitamin that pregnant women are urged to take because it prevents neural tube defects. Researchers first began to link folate deficiency with depression in the 1960s, and we've since come to understand that people with depression tend to be deficient in this vitamin. Increasing levels can alleviate symptoms. But the primary supplemental form is folic acid (used in both B-complex vitamins and fortified foods), which is synthetic and not processed by the body in the same way as natural folate is. Research shows that there are many benefits to using the natural form of folate (5-methyltetrahydrofolate) because it is better absorbed, it does not mask B_{12} deficiency as easily, and it helps avoid the pitfalls of unmetabolized folic acid in circulation, which has been associated with an increased risk of cancer.[6]

Vitamin B_{12} comes in a few different forms, which vary in efficacy and safety. Cyanocobalamin is the most commonly used form of the nutrient. It's less expensive, but it is not found in nature, and its metabolism may release small amounts of cyanide into the system. That's right: cyanide. While this could never be enough to cause cyanide poisoning, it's a potential issue for people who have impaired detox as a result of genetic issues, nutrient deficiencies, or chronic illness. The most desirable form of B_{12} is methylcobalamin, which is the form produced by our gut bacteria.

So when you're looking for a B complex, make sure it contains folate as 5-methyltetrahydrofolate or folinic acid and B_{12} as methylcobalamin (or hydroxocobalamin or adenosylcobalamin) in addition to the other B vitamins. I am partial to replacement of B_{12} by injection because it is a foolproof method. This treatment consists of 1 to 5 milligrams administered one to five times weekly for two to four weeks, depending on an individual's circumstances and response. For some patients, it's the last antidepressant they ever need.

Minerals

Magnesium, zinc, iodine, and selenium are essential to the body's functionality. Each one of these has been specifically studied for its impact on mood. Magnesium deficiency, for example, is found in 80 percent of depressed individuals, and may play a strong role in anxiety by disrupting the body's HPA axis (the stress response system).[7,8] And we've long documented low levels of magnesium in the cerebral spinal fluid of suicidal patients.[9]

Although we used to get plenty of minerals through foods, most of us are deficient today as a result of both modern farming practices that deplete the soil of these elements and processing techniques. Low mineral levels can also be caused by high sugar consumption. This makes simple carbohydrates like bread, cake, and cookies doubly problematic—not only do they fail to provide good-quality nutrients, but they also dysregulate blood sugar and further deplete minerals from the body. Look for a multimineral supplement that contains a collection of minerals. Take your minerals with food, as some can cause gastric upset. These are my recommendations:

MAGNESIUM

Typical dosages range from 150 to 800 milligrams a day. In patients with more prominent anxiety, insomnia, and premenstrual symptoms I focus on doses higher than 300 milligrams a day. I usually recommend magnesium glycinate over other types, unless there is a problem with constipation; magnesium citrate and magnesium oxide provide a nice laxative side benefit.

ZINC

This essential "resiliency" mineral plays a part in controlling the brain and body's response to stress; in fact, three hundred or more enzymes in our bodies require zinc to conduct their functions, including making DNA, protein synthesis, and cell division. Zinc is also critical to cell signaling. The highest amount of zinc in the body is found in our brains, particularly in the memory part of our brains called the hippocampus. Zinc deficiency has been shown to lead to symptoms of depression, ADHD, difficulties with learning and memory, seizures, aggression, and violence. Optimal zinc dosage is 15 to 30 milligrams a day, and zinc gluconate is an optimal form. Copper is an essential complementary nutrient, with a typical dose of 1 to 3 milligrams daily.

IODINE

Iodine plays a critical role in the formation of thyroid hormone. Soil depletion and exposure to chemicals that interfere with iodine incorporation in the body, from bromine in processed foods and flame retardants to chlorine and fluoride in water, prevent us from getting enough iodine. Iodine can be obtained through uncontaminated sea vegetables, eggs, and supplementation in the 200 microgram to 3 milligram range. I recommend starting with a supplement that contains Atlantic kelp.

SELENIUM

Selenium is a mineral essential for replenishing glutathione, a master antioxidant in the body, by acting as a cofactor for the enzyme glutathione peroxidase, the enzyme that helps make glutathione. Due to soil erosion, it is notoriously absent in modern food. Mass market forms like sodium selenite can be toxic, so always opt for a chelated form, preferably selenomethionine or selenium glycinate.

Selenium supports neurologic function, helps the body produce mood-lifting neurotransmitters, and is especially important in the conversion of the thyroid hormone thyroxine (T4) to its more active form triiodothyronine (T3). One review looked at five studies, all of which indicated that low selenium intake is associated with poor mood.[10] Studies supplementing with selenium revealed that selenium improved mood and diminished anxiety.[11] This is remarkable when you consider just how infinitesimal a therapeutic dose is. As low as 200 micrograms can do the trick, and that's only one-fifth of a milligram (which is only one thousandth of a gram)!

Typical dosage of selenium is 100 to 200 μg a day. Selenium is ideal for anxious and depressive individuals who also have low thyroid function and/or low T3 levels.

Fatty acids

Fatty acids are essential to the structure and function of cell membranes. Without them, cells would simply fall apart. Cellular membranes are lipid envelopes that encase and protect the internal workings of cells. There are more than 100 trillion cells in the human body, all with the same basic membrane structure, even for the neurons of our brain that carry all of our messages to and fro. The membrane is essential for the production of energy in the mitochondria, for without the double membrane structure there is no storage space for the separation of an electrical charge—no way of conducting chemical reactions to create energy. The volume of cellular membrane in the body is mind-boggling. The liver alone has more than 300,000 square feet of membrane, the equivalent of more than four and a half football fields!

From my personal research and clinical work with patients, I've found that the best way to obtain supplemental fatty acids is to focus on natural fats and take supplements that add more omega-3 and omega-6 fatty acids. Fish and cod liver oil supplements contain two superstar omega-3 fatty acids—eicosapentaenoic acid (EPA) and docosahexaenoic acid (DHA). These fatty acids have been shown to reduce inflammation and boost brain regeneration.

A number of studies support the use of fish oil for depression and anxiety.[12] A typical therapeutic dosage of fish oil is 1 to 2 grams of EPA with DHA in a three to two ratio. Read the fish oil label closely—if it does not break down the numbers, then purchase one that does. Because of the poor environmental stewardship of our seas, fish are at risk of high contaminant levels from mercury and other metals, dioxins, PCBs, and more. Make sure to purchase fish oil from a trusted company (see the Resources page on my website). The best companies use a process of filtration known as molecular distillation, which prevents rancidity and ensures that the oil is certified contaminant free. You can also find some sources that are extracted using nontoxic carbon dioxide at high pressure, or a low-temperature extraction called supercritical extraction.

EVENING PRIMROSE OIL

Extracted from the seeds of its namesake wildflower, evening primrose offers a rich source of omega-6 fatty acids, specifically the anti-inflammatory omega-6 gamma-linolenic acid (GLA), which is hard to come by in the diet. For the past nearly one hundred years, evening primrose has been used to address a wide variety of health problems, from brittle nails and hair, eczema, premenstrual syndrome, and menopausal symptoms to rheumatoid arthritis, multiple sclerosis, and neurological disorders. Look for high-quality oil certified as organic, and start with 500 milligrams twice daily.

COD LIVER OIL

Oil from the liver of Atlantic cod has helped humankind for centuries. It has been used as a fuel for lamps, in the tanning of hides, in liquid soaps, as a base for paint, and, most important, as food and therapy. Cod liver oil is a nutritional powerhouse and was once a standard supplement in traditional European societies. Weston Price recommended that cod liver oil be taken with vitamin K2–rich butter oil to complement the naturally occurring fat-soluble vitamins in cod liver oil. It's not only a rich source of the omega fatty acids EPA and DHA, it also includes naturally occurring vitamins A and D and can be a great alternative to fish oil, which lacks these vitamins. Its vitamin D content has made it famous for preventing and curing vitamin D deficiency and its horrid consequences at the extreme: rickets. You'll want to find a cod liver oil supplement that hasn't been stripped of its vitamins and contains a five to one ratio of vitamin A to vitamin D. Look for a naturally produced cod liver oil made using a filtering process that retains the natural vitamins and ideally is packaged in a nitrogen-flushed glass bottle. Aim for a supplement with at least 2500 IUs of vitamin A and 250 IUs of vitamin D per teaspoon.[13]

ADRENAL AND HYPOTHALAMUS GLANDULARS

Glandular supplements, also commonly called glandulars, are made from various organs and tissues of mammals. They were used successfully to treat multiple conditions throughout the nineteenth and early twentieth centuries. They have recently been making a comeback, thanks to new science showing their positive effects on damaged tissues and organs by exposing the tissues to growth factors that influence the body's capacity for self-repair and regeneration. Because glandulars contain a complex array of enzymes, vitamins, fatty acids, amino acids, minerals, and neurotransmitters and a host of nutrients in addition to the tissues within the gland, they are difficult to study in a standardized way. On the other hand, this also makes them a food, and one that we are increasingly finding to be far more beneficial to our physiology than the sum of its parts can convey.

Adrenal cortex is most helpful for depressive symptoms in addition to a general adrenal glandular. Adrenals must come from pastured animals. Begin with one twice daily of each.

Hypothalamus is a calming glandular that begins to repair the communication between the brain and glands. Take one to four for agitation and acute anxiety along with one twice daily. Over time, you will need less.

DIGESTIVE ENZYMES

If your body doesn't generate enough digestive enzymes, you can't break down your food, so even if you're eating well, you aren't absorbing all that good nutrition. You'll also put excess burden on the available enzymes being used to digest your food, taking them away from their other role of maintaining and healing your body. That's when supplemental digestive enzymes come into play, especially while you're rehabilitating your gut and restoring optimal digestive function. Enzyme therapy is based on the work of Dr. Edward Howell in the 1920s and 1930s. Howell proposed that enzymes from foods work in the stomach to predigest food. By cooking foods, many of these enzymes are denatured while digestibility is enhanced. Supplementation with plant-based enzymes is complemented by animal-based enzymes such as those found in pancreas glandulars.

There are a variety of digestive enzymes on the market. Look for ones that come from plant sources and contain a mix of enzymes, including proteases (which break down proteins), lipases (which break down fats), and amylase (which breaks down carbohydrates). Some formulas include a variety of each type of enzyme operating at different pH ranges so that they will work with every individual and various food combinations. Dr. Nicholas Gonzalez brought the relevance of pancreatic enzymes into the management of chronic disease and advised supplementing with extremely high quality pancreas glandulars, which is my preferred way of complementing plant-based enzymes for digestive support. Take one to three high-quality digestive enzymes and pancreas glandulars within thirty minutes of a meal.

BETAINE HCL

To boost your stomach's ability to digest food, betaine hydrochloride is your friend—especially if your stomach doesn't produce enough acid, which is an all too common problem. Betaine HCL is an acidic form of betaine, a vitamin-like substance found in some foods. It increases the level of hydrochloric acid in the stomach necessary for proper digestion and assimilation of nutrients from food. People with heartburn, indigestion, gas, and reflux are often told that their stomachs are producing too much acid, but that's a common misconception reinforced by conventional medicine, which routinely prescribes stomach acid–blocking medications at the slightest sign of stomach dysfunction. It fails to properly diagnose the digestive problem, which is often the opposite: too little acid, which results in the putrefaction of food that releases irritating and ulcer-causing gases such as hydrogen sulfide. This mimics excess HCL but is actually caused by a deficiency. One to three capsules (one is typically around 500 mg) with each protein-containing meal is a typical dose. You will likely require less after one to two months. If you have a heartburn sensation with as little as one capsule, this supplement is not for you.

Additional Supplements to Consider

SAMe

SAMe, a naturally occurring molecule synthesized by the one-carbon cycle that is dependent on B_{12} and folate, is a precursor to many key biomolecules including creatine, phosphatidylcholine, co-enzyme Q10, carnitine, and myelin. All of these chemicals in the body play a role in pain, depression, liver disease, and other conditions. SAMe also participates in the production of neurotransmitters and has been approved as a nutraceutical since the 1990s and prescribed in Europe for depression for three decades. Numerous double-blind studies have proven its efficacy for depression and anxiety.[14] Try 400 to 1,600 milligrams daily; look for capsules that are enteric coated and packaged into a blister pack.

L-THEANINE

L-theanine is a calming amino acid found primarily in tea. It can promote alpha wave brain production, which can reduce anxiety and support a relaxed but focused mind-set. It's like meditation in a capsule! Start with 1 to 200 milligrams twice daily.

N-ACETYL CYSTEINE (NAC)

N-acetyl cysteine is a slightly modified version of the sulfur-containing amino acid cysteine. When taken as a supplement, NAC replenishes intracellular levels of the natural antioxidant glutathione (GSH), helping to restore the ability of cells to fight damage from free radicals. Much of NAC's beneficial activity comes from its capacity to control the expression of genes related to the inflammatory response; it has also been shown to improve insulin sensitivity and to be effective for treating compulsive behaviors. Aim for 600 to 1800 milligrams a day. Clinical studies have found that doses of up to 2000 milligrams a day are safe and effective.

RHODIOLA

Rhodiola rosea, sometimes called Arctic root or golden root, is an adaptogenic herb—it acts in nonspecific ways to increase resistance to stress without disrupting normal biological functions. Evidence suggests that it's an antioxidant with the ability to boost immune system function, and can even increase athletic and sexual energy. The herb grows at high altitudes in the arctic areas of Europe and Asia, and its root has been used in traditional medicine in Russia and Scandinavia for centuries. A study published in 2007 showed that patients with mild to moderate depression who took a rhodiola extract reported fewer symptoms of depression than those who took a placebo.[15] A small human trial of the herb at UCLA published in 2008 reported significant improvement in ten people with generalized anxiety who took the herb for ten weeks.[16] So go ahead and try some: start with 100 milligrams once a day for a week and then increase the dosage by 100 milligrams every week, up to 400 milligrams a day. And seek products that contain 2 to 3 percent rosavin and 0.8 to 1 percent salidroside.

CURCUMIN

I've written a lot about curcumin—what I've called the wonder drug that works—in my blog posts. The medical literature exploring the efficacy of curcumin—the most active polyphenol in the Indian spice turmeric—continues to explode, with more than seven thousand published studies available today. Curcumin is both a therapeutic agent used in a spectrum of health conditions and nature's anti-inflammatory. It's also a potent antioxidant and neuroprotective agent, hormonal and neurochemical modulator, and a general friend to our genome.[17] Unless you're cooking with a lot of it, try it in supplement form: 500 to 1000 milligrams twice daily.

PROBIOTICS

Although you'll be getting lots of natural probiotics (and what good bacteria love to eat—prebiotics, which is resistant starch and fiber) from your new dietary protocol, it doesn't hurt to add more probiotics via a supplement. The strains that have been demonstrated to influence the immune system include *L. paracasei, L. rhamnosus, L. acidophilus, L. johnsonii, L. fermentum, L. reuteri, L. plantarum, B. longum,* and *B. animalis.* The best studied for anti-inflammatory functions are *L. paracasei, L. plantarum, and P. pentosaceus.* The ones I've highlighted in bold have been shown to potentially have pharmaceutical-like effects in some studies.[18] Strains in the *Bifidobacterium* and *Lactobacillus* genuses have an emerging role in psychiatric treatment and are readily available in commercial products. Look for high-quality probiotics that contain a variety of strains in the billions (see the Resources page on my website). Take daily according to the dosage on the label.

If You're Tapering from an SSRI

I'll offer more specifics on this protocol in Chapter 10, but I highly recommend considering a broad spectrum amino acid supplement as well as a high-quality tryptophan or 5-HTP supplement. Because more research is needed to optimize dosing schedule and amounts, a good place to start would be 500 milligrams a day of tryptophan taken with a simple carbohydrate (a slice of apple or a gluten-free cracker) on an empty stomach and work up to 3 grams a day if needed. Dosages of 5-HTP can start at 50 milligrams three times a day and work up to 200 milligrams three times a day, also taken on an empty stomach. The complementary amino acid tyrosine is important if you are taking tryptophan or 5-HTP for more than a few weeks (1500 milligrams two to four times daily before meals). Inositol, pharmaGaba, or phenibut can also be helpful calming agents during this time. In my experience, specific amino acids are only necessary during the medication taper.

If You're Thinking About Bioidentical Hormones

If you know that your symptoms are linked to your period in intensity and/or frequency, start with maca and progress to chaste tree. Maca is a root that belongs to the radish family and is grown in the mountains of Peru; it is also known as Peruvian ginseng. Maca's benefits have been long valued; the root was prized throughout the Incan empire for its adaptogenic-like qualities that enable it to nourish and balance the body's delicate hormonal system and to help cope with stress. It also energizes naturally, without the adverse side effects of caffeine, and it can aid in reproductive function, helping to balance hormones and increase fertility. Maca is most commonly available in powder form. In my practice I use a particular gelatinized product by Natural Health International and dose according to the recommendations on the label with great success.

Chaste tree (Vitex agnus-castus)

Chaste tree has been widely used by European and North American herbalists to treat acne, digestive complaints, menstrual irregularities, premenstrual syndrome (PMS), and infertility, and also for lactation support. Vitex is a deciduous shrub native to European, Mediterranean, and Central Asian countries; its berries have been used medically for centuries. Its hormone balancing powers make it an ideal natural aid in combating conditions related to the menstrual cycle, from irregularities to menopause.[19,20,21] A standard dose is between 150 to 250 milligrams containing 30 to 40 milligrams of dried fruit extract.

Inositol

When blood sugar imbalances are at the root of menstrual irregularity (think polycystic ovarian syndrome), the carbohydrate molecule myo-inositol is a multitasker. It improves insulin sensitivity, reduces male hormones (at dosages of 2 to 4 grams daily), and has even been studied for anxiety and obsessive compulsive symptoms (at dosages of 12 to 18 grams daily).[22,23,24] There is some evidence that combining myo-inositol and d-chiro-inositol in a forty to one ratio is most effective for hormone rebalancing.[25]

SUPPLEMENTAL DEVICES

While I am most interested in root-cause resolution of what we are calling depression and anxiety resulting from food intolerances, sugar imbalance, thyroid autoimmunity, nutrient deficiency, and stress, I often present my patients with alternative options for more immediate symptom relief. I have been prescribing the Fisher Wallace Cranial Electrical Stimulator (CES), a device that generates a low-intensity alternating current that is transmitted across the skull, for many years now (I have no financial relationship with this company). I have come to think of it as meditation in a gadget. It was cleared by the FDA in 1979 and works from the premise that we are energetic beings and that accessing the body's ability to recalibrate can come in many different forms. The recommendation is to use it for twenty minutes twice daily to promote alpha wave activity and to modulate neurotransmitters, endorphins, and cortisol.[26] My patients who try it typically use it regularly for three weeks and then as needed.

With more than 160 published human studies including twenty-three randomized controlled trials reporting positive results, it's curious that I never learned about this extremely low-risk treatment option in my decade of training. A newer study published in 2014 added to the growing body of evidence: two scientists used a five-week randomized, double-blind, placebo-controlled design to test the effectiveness of CES treatment on various anxiety disorders and depression within a primary care setting.[27] A breathtaking 83 percent of patients experienced a reduction of more than 50 percent of their symptoms of depression relative to controls in a matter of weeks. And 82 percent of those with anxiety experienced the same relief. See the Resource section for information on how to obtain this device.

Another nifty gadget I recommend to my patients, especially those who have trouble with sleep, is a light box. As the body has its own internal clock set by the cycles of day and night, the ideal way to reset an upset body clock is to expose yourself to bright morning sunlight. This ties directly into our physiology and how we feel. Receptors at the backs of your eyes capture the light and send messages to the brain to recalibrate your clock. Light boxes produce artificial light that mimics the sun's intensity without emitting ultraviolet radiation. They are designed to produce those perfect wavelengths of light (peaking in the optimal "blue" wavelength range, or 460 nanometers) with the light directed to your eyes at an angle for the greatest effect. See the Resources page on my website for more information on light boxes.

GARGLE POWER

Dr. Datis Kharrazian, a functional neurologist and author of *Why Isn't My Brain Working?*, has synthesized vast bodies of research and contributed cutting-edge solutions to the realm of cognitive impairment and degenerative conditions. One of his recommendations to activate the vagus nerve and to stimulate gut-brain harmony and improve gut motility is simple and effective: fill a glass of water and gargle forcefully with each sip until your eyes tear. Do this several times a day.

SUPPORT TEAM

While I believe that a doctor's role is to share the tools for self-healing with a patient, I also believe in finding your healing team. I am an avid supporter of a variety of practitioners and refer widely. Many of my patients have made astronomical leaps and bounds in their health through the work of craniosacral therapists, neurofeedback specialists, and acupuncturists and through energy medicine modalities from sound healing to bodywork to homeopathy.

I believe that energy medicine is the medicine of the future.

All forms of healing in history have honored mind, body, and spirit. Science is catching up, however, and quantum physics has already begun to explain the informational capacity of subatomic energy, the limitations of quantification, and the relevance of systems and networks. Energy medicine acknowledges that, fundamentally, our existence on this planet is attributable to unseen and poorly understood forces. These forces can be awakened and harnessed for spontaneous healing. In fact, as stated by the great twentieth-century philosopher Alan Watts, the Chinese word for nature means *that which happens of itself*. Nature cannot be commanded or forced to comply, without consequence. Energy medicine does not rely on fallible beliefs about biology, the latest, greatest paper, nor the reigning trend in combating disease. It relies simply on the gifts of healers who can unlock the body's natural potential. It's simple, elegant, and powerful, and it puts us back in touch with our most fundamental driver—that chi, prana, shakti, or whatever word we use to describe that undeniable vital force that infuses our body with life and our mind with clarity and ease.

'TWAS THE NIGHT BEFORE

Take a deep breath. I've given you a lot of information so far. You've learned more about the habits of a woman who lives on a natural high than most practicing doctors and psychiatrists today. If you haven't already begun to make some of the changes I've recommended, now is your chance. With the next chapter, you'll follow a four-week program designed to shift your diet and rehabilitate your body and brain back to optimal well-being. You'll arrive at a place where you feel energetic and emotionally vibrant. It's the place we all dream of being—and it's much closer than you think.

Making lifestyle changes, even small ones, can seem overwhelming at first. You wonder how you can avoid falling back onto your usual habits. Will you feel deprived and hungry? Will you find it impossible to keep up this new lifestyle forever? Is this program doable given the time you have and the commitments you've already made? And can you reach a point where following these guidelines is second nature?

This program is the answer. It's a simple, straightforward strategy that has the right balance of structure and adaptability to honor your personal preferences and power of choice. You will finish my four-week program with the knowledge and inspiration to stay on a healthy path for the rest of your life. The closer you stick to my guidelines, the faster you will see results. Bear in mind that this program has many benefits beyond the obvious physical ones. Ending depression might be first and foremost on your mind, but the rewards don't end there. You will see change in every area of your life. You will feel more confident and have more self-esteem. You'll feel younger and more in control of your life and future. You'll be able to navigate through stressful times with ease, have the motivation to stay active and engage with others, and feel more accomplished at work and home. In short, you will feel and *be* more productive and fulfilled. And your success will breed more success. When your life becomes richer, fuller, and more energized as a result of your efforts, you won't want to revert to your old unhealthy lifestyle. I know you can do this. You must, for yourself and your loved ones. The payoffs—and the potentially calamitous consequences if you don't—are huge.

So get yourself oriented for the next chapter of your life. For the reset you didn't think was possible. For the roof to blow off of your expectations for your experience in this life. Get ready to shift and to watch the changes be delivered to you.

To start, on the night before your thirty days, take nineteen minutes to try the following exercise. It's a kriya (yogic series) that can powerfully take the garbage out from your cluttered mind and infuse your path with potential.* Read the instructions once through, then use a timer for each of the three parts. It goes like this:

Part One: Sitting in easy pose (cross-legged on the floor or on a chair with your feet flat on the floor), stretch the spine up straight and close your eyes. Hands rest on your knees with the tip of your index finger touching your thumb on each hand (this is called Gyan Mudra). Drink the breath in in a single long sip through a rounded mouth. Then close the mouth and exhale through the nose slowly and completely. Continue for 7 minutes.

Part Two: Inhale and hold the breath comfortably. As you hold the breath in, meditate on zero. Think to yourself: "All is zero; I am zero; each thought is zero; my pain is zero; that problem is zero; that illness is zero." Meditate on all negative or emotional mental and physical conditions and situations, and as each comes to mind, bring it to zero—a single point of light, a small, insignificant nonexistence. Exhale and repeat for 7 minutes, breathing in a comfortable rhythm.

Part Three: Think of the quality or condition you most desire for your complete happiness and growth. Summarize it in a single word such as "wealth," "health," "relationship," "guidance," "knowledge," "luck." Lock on to this single word and visualize the

---

* This exercise and others can be found at http://www.spiritvoyage.com and http://www.yogibhajan.org

various facets of it. Experience how it feels to have this quality or condition in your life now. Inhale and suspend the breath as you beam the thought in a continuous stream. Lock on to it. Relax the breath as needed and repeat for 5 minutes.

To End:
Inhale and gently shake out your shoulders, arms, and spine. Then stretch your arms up, spread your fingers wide, and breathe deeply a few times.

Now you're ready to turn the page . . .

CHAPTER 10

4 Weeks to a Natural High

A 30-Day Plan of Action

Welcome to a new, wonderful you.

This past June, a woman I'll call Jane e-mailed me from abroad, where she's been living with her husband and four children (under the age of ten!). She wrote:

Here is my dilemma . . . I normally would just "suck it up" and wait it out, but my issues are seriously impeding my quality of life. I've had Hashimoto's for many years now and anxiety even longer. I've experienced significant GI symptoms since 2011 when I was treated for H. pylori. I can no longer tolerate gluten, but eliminating it from my diet hasn't eradicated the bloating, discomfort, fatigue, etc. I take oral contraceptives to help regulate PMS, which was particularly problematic after the birth of my kids. When my anxiety worsened and I developed major insomnia, I saw a psychiatrist, who prescribed Zoloft, which I took for two years. I gained weight despite running 15 to 20 miles per week, one of the things that helps me considerably. I changed to Pristiq, which I did not like after trying it for about three months. I felt jittery, sweaty, and dizzy much of the day. I am now off those meds. I don't know how much of an appreciable difference they made in the first place.

Jane's experience reflects that of so many of the women who reach out to me searching desperately for a cure. She came to see me within weeks of writing this e-mail, and I prescribed a protocol that I felt confident would garner results within a month. It's the same protocol that you will find in this chapter; I'll take you step-by-step for the next four weeks to help you put what you've learned from me into action—no matter what kind of psychiatric diagnosis you already have or hope to avoid. You'll learn how to execute the changes you need to make in your daily lifestyle choices.

You might be panicking at the thought of losing some of your favorite foods. I realize that for some people ditching bread, pasta, pizza, pastries, and most desserts (among other things) is going to be tough. Change is hard. And changing long-established habits is harder. I am often asked right off the bat, "What am I going to *eat*?" Without even bringing to mind a potential taper from meds in your future (after the first thirty days; see page 267), you may be worrying about withdrawal from sugar and wheat. And what if you have an insatiable desire for carbs? Perhaps you're anticipating colossal cravings that you won't be able to resist, fearing the body's reaction to a dietary U-turn. If willpower isn't in your vocabulary, you may be wondering if this is truly doable.

Well, let me be the first to say that yes—all of this is possible. You just need to take the initial plunge. Within a matter of days or a couple of weeks I predict that you'll have fewer anxious thoughts, better sleep, and improved energy. You'll feel clearer, lighter, and more resilient to your daily stressors. Over time, you'll likely watch unwanted weight fall off too, and specific laboratory tests will show vast improvements in many areas of your biochemistry.

It's a good idea to check with your doctor about beginning this new program, especially if you have serious health issues such as diabetes. This is important if you're going to opt for some of my "turbo-charge" strategies like the coffee enema or bentonite clay; if you're currently taking meds and hope to wean yourself, commit to the first thirty days, and then I'll give you additional instructions on page 267.

Over the course of the next month, you will achieve four important goals:

1. Introduce a new way of nourishing your body through the foods you eat.
2. Green your home and environment, divorcing yourself from the modern love affair with toxicants.
3. Incorporate a daily meditative practice into your life, one that stimulates the body's natural relaxation response and paves the way for lasting transformation.
4. Prioritize getting routine restful sleep and adequate exercise throughout the week.

I've broken down the program into four weeks, with each week devoted to focusing on one of these specific goals so you can establish a new rhythm and maintain these healthy habits for life. In the days leading up to the first week, you should consider seeing your doctor to have the tests I outlined in Chapter 9 performed to establish your baseline. You'll also use this time to get your kitchen organized and begin to wean yourself from sugar and wheat products as you clear out the junk and replace it with real whole foods.

During week 1, "Dietary Detox," you'll start my menu plan and execute my nutritional recommendations, which you'll continue throughout the thirty days.

During week 2, "Home Detox," I'll encourage you to green your home and living environment and try some detox strategies like skin brushing and a coffee enema.

In week 3, "Peace of Mind," you'll turn your attention to establishing a daily meditative practice to switch on your body's natural relaxation response. This will become a daily habit for life.

During week 4, "Movement and Sleep," you'll start a regular workout program if you haven't done so already. I'll give you ideas for moving more throughout the day. I'll also be asking you to focus on your sleep habits and follow a few simple guidelines to ensure that you're achieving the best sleep possible every single night, weekends included.

I'll be helping you put all the elements of this program together and equipping you with strategies for permanently establishing these new behaviors in your life. Don't second-guess your ability to succeed; I've designed this program to be as practical and easy to follow as possible.

PRELUDE TO WEEK 1: PREPARE

Determine Your Baseline

Prior to beginning the dietary program, have the following laboratory studies performed in addition to routine blood and urine tests, if possible. Use the information in Chapter 9 to learn how to understand target levels and results.

- ▸ TSH, free T3, free T4 *Is your thyroid sick?*
- ▸ Thyroid autoantibodies, reverse T3
- ▸ MTHFR gene variant *Do you carry a mutation?*
- ▸ Vitamin B_{12}, homocysteine *Are you B_{12} deficient?*
- ▸ High-sensitivity C-reactive protein *What are your inflammation levels?*
- ▸ Hemoglobin A1C *How balanced is your blood sugar?*
- ▸ Vitamin D *Are you deficient in D?*

Upon completion of the four-week program, you may opt to have your stool tested to further detect imbalances in your gut microbiome. A salivary cortisol test and, if indicated, a urinary organic acid test may also be in order depending on your unique circumstances. If your baseline tests show that you're deficient in vitamins for which supplementation is recommended, by all means you can consider starting those supplements on day one. Otherwise, hold off on starting any supplement regimen until the beginning of the third week. That's when you can begin to add the core basics (listed below) into your daily menu, and customize your regimen with additional supplements (also listed below) as needed after the thirty days.

Kitchen Cleanup

In the days leading up to your new way of eating, you'll want to take inventory of your kitchen and eliminate items that you'll no longer be eating. Start by removing the following:

▸ All sources of gluten (see page 150 for the full list), including whole-grain and whole wheat bread, noodles, pasta, pastries, baked goods, and cereals.

▸ All forms of processed carbs, sugar, and packaged foods: chips, crackers, cookies, pastries, muffins, pizza dough, cake, dough-nuts, sugary snacks, candy, energy bars, ice cream/frozen yogurt/sherbet, jams/jellies/preserves, ketchup, processed cheese spreads, juices, dried fruit, sports drinks, soft drinks/ soda, fried foods, sugar (white and brown), and corn syrup.

▸ Margarine, vegetable shortening, and commercial brands of cooking oil (soybean, corn, cottonseed, canola, peanut, saf-flower, grapeseed, sunflower, rice bran, and wheat germ oils)— even if they are organic.

▸ Dairy (including butter, milk, yogurt, cheese, cream, and ice cream) and soy (including soy milk, soy cheese, soy burgers, soy hot dogs, soy ice cream, soy yogurt, soy sauce, and any-thing that has "soy protein isolate" on the list of ingredients).

Then restock. The following items can be consumed liberally (go organic and local with your whole-food choices wherever possible):

▸ **Healthy fats:** Extra-virgin olive oil, organic virgin coconut oil, red palm oil, grass-fed and organic or pasture-fed ghee, flax oil, macadamia nut oil, avocado, coconut, olives, nuts and nut butters, lard, tallow, and seeds (flax seeds, sunflower seeds, pumpkin seeds, sesame seeds, chia seeds).

▸ **Herbs, seasonings, and condiments:** There are virtually no restrictions on herbs and seasonings so long as they are fresh, organic, and free of dyes and artificial colorings. Toss out your ketchup and any condiment that's laced with gluten, soy, and sugar or that's been processed in a plant with wheat and soy. It's fine to enjoy mustard, horseradish, tapenade, guacamole, and salsa if they are free of processed ingredients.

▸ **Whole fruit and vegetables:** See Chapter 6 for lists.

▸ **Protein:** Whole pastured eggs; wild fish; shellfish and mollusks; grass-fed meat, fowl, poultry, and pork; wild game (see Chapter 6 for lists).

WEEK 1: DIETARY DETOX

Now that your kitchen is in order, it's time to learn how to prepare your meals. On page 252, you'll find a day-by-day menu plan for the first week; this will serve as a model for planning your meals for the remaining three weeks. Unlike other diets, this one won't ask you to count calories, limit fat intake, or fret over portion sizes. There is no portion control; portion control happens naturally, with you eating until you're satisfied. Pay attention to when you're hungry, as you'll find your appetite shifting over the weeks. The good news is that this type of diet is enormously self-regulating— you won't find yourself overeating, and you'll feel full for several hours before needing another meal.

When your body is running mostly on sugar, it's being driven by the glucose-insulin roller-coaster ride that triggers intense hunger when your blood sugar plunges, followed by short-lived satiety. Eating a low-sugar, higher-fat diet will have the opposite effect. By providing a cleaner and more efficient source of steady energy, it will eliminate cravings and prevent those mental shutdowns in the late afternoon that can happen on sugar-based diets. It will automatically allow you to control calories without even thinking about it, burn more fat, put an end to mindless eating (those extra 500 calories or so a day many people unconsciously consume to bail out blood sugar chaos), and effortlessly boost your body's overall performance. And when your pancreas is no longer constantly forced to produce extra insulin, those of you struggling with weight issues may see those extra hard-to-lose pounds rapidly melt off. Say goodbye to feeling moody, foggy, sluggish, and tired throughout the day. And say hello to a whole new you.

The only difference between this month and beyond is that you're going to also eliminate all dairy, grains (except quinoa and buckwheat), white rice, white potatoes, corn, and beans. I'll show you how to invite these foods back into your diet in moderation on page 264. You might find it helpful to keep a food journal throughout the program. Make notes about recipes you like and foods that you think might still be giving you trouble (example: you experience symptoms such as joint pain or brain fogginess every time you eat sweet bell peppers).

Avoid eating out during the first two weeks, so you can focus on getting the dietary protocol down. This will prepare you for when you do eat outside of your home and need to make good decisions about what to order. The first two weeks will work to eliminate your cravings, so there will be less temptation when you're looking at a menu filled with mood-busting foods.

During week 1, focus on mastering your new eating habits. Use my recipes, including my sample seven-day meal plan, or venture out on your own as long as you stick to the guidelines. If you follow the first week's plan, configuring your own meals in the future will be a cinch.

When you're strapped for time and don't have access to a kitchen, which is often the case for lunch, pack food. Having precooked foods or foods prepared in advance—such as roasted or broiled chicken, poached salmon, bone broth, or strips of grilled sirloin steak—in your refrigerator ready to go is helpful. Packets of nuts and seeds and cans of sardines are handy to have around. Fill a container with salad greens and chopped raw veggies and add meat, fish, or an egg and some olive oil to bring with you. And don't forget about leftovers. Many of the recipes can be made over the weekend (and doubled to make more) to cover multiple meals during the week.

What to Drink: Nothing but Pure, Filtered Water Over the Next Thirty Days

Drink half of your body weight in ounces of water daily. If you weigh 150 pounds, that means drinking at least 75 ounces, or about nine glasses (8 ounces each) of pure water (no tap!) per day. No alcohol, coffee, tea, soda, or fruit drinks of any kind. Some may need to wean off of caffeinated beverages such as coffee using increasing portions of organic decaf varieties for a week prior to initiating the program. Then it's just water, water, water because all other beverages including tea have diuretic effects and replace vital water intake. After thirty days, you may bring alcohol, coffee, and tea back (see page 265). I recommend that you begin your day with two glasses of water; add a tablespoon of apple cider vinegar if you like for its acidifying effects—a key nutritional tool for depression according to Dr. Gonzalez. Then drink one full glass of water between meals.

In the past decade, there's been a huge shift in the variety of food available at our markets. If you live in an urban area, for instance, you're likely to be able to purchase any kind of ingredient within a matter of miles, whether that means visiting your usual grocery store, which now likely has a good selection of organic foods, or venturing to a local farmers' market. Get to know your grocers; they can tell you what just came in and where your foods are coming from. Aim for choosing produce that's in season, and be willing to try new foods like fermented vegetables and sardines (if you like canned tuna, you'll love them, I promise!). Go organic or wild whenever possible—choosing quality over cost has incalculable benefits. When in doubt, ask your grocer.

As you are eliminating addictive foods like alcohol, sugar, refined carbs, and dairy, you will have an opportunity to relate to food in a totally different way. You will no longer be at the beck and call of your cravings, using food as reward and punishment, and thinking about it all day long. When you eat, it will taste good, satisfy hunger by nourishing you deeply, and keep you feeling stable. Exactly what food is meant to do!

What kind of cheats would sabotage the whole month? I am an absolutist about this first phase because there's nothing worse than ambiguous results. No one wants to feel tortured by a diet for thirty days, only to get to the end without feeling all of the benefits of the full plan. Choose a thirty-day window to set yourself up to succeed. January through April can be good times of the year with fewer commitments for many people. There are some cheats that will force a restart of the month, in particular gluten and dairy (including soy sauce and butter, for example). This means that if you go out to a restaurant, you will treat yourself like a celiac and lactose intolerant patient and ask your waiter for gluten- and dairy-free options. These days most restaurants are familiar with these restrictions. And this is a great litmus test for a good restaurant: restaurants that are aware are generally more concerned about the quality and freshness of what they serve. In my experience, a bite or even a serving of corn or soy, beans, rice, or even a glass of alcohol will not require a reset, but do your best to clear the slate.

SNACKS

Because the meals on my plan are highly satisfying and blood-sugar-stabilizing, you're not likely to find yourself ravenously hunting for food in between meals after the first ten to fourteen days. But it's nice to know that you can snack whenever you need to. Here are some ideas:

▶ A handful of raw nuts and/or seeds (preferably sprouted, and no peanuts)

▶ A few squares of authentic dark chocolate that doesn't contain any white sugar (anything 70 percent cacao and above)

▶ Chopped raw vegetables (such as bell peppers, broccoli, cucumber, or radishes) dipped in guacamole, tapenade, or nut butter

▶ Roasted turkey or roast beef slices or chicken slices dipped in mustard

▶ Half an avocado with olive oil, lemon, salt, and pepper

▶ Two soft-boiled eggs

▶ Berries with coconut milk (unsweetened, full-fat)

▶ Bone broth

▶ Grass-fed jerky

▶ Lactofermented vegetables

▶ Seaweed (Atlantic is preferable)

SAMPLE MENU FOR A WEEK

Here is what a typical week will look like. Recipes are highlighted in boldface; the recipe section begins on page 281. Note: you can use organic extra-virgin olive oil, grass-fed ghee, or virgin coconut oil for sautéing, and avoid processed oils and cooking sprays unless the spray is made from organic olive oil. The most important part of the first thirty days is to exclude all grains (especially gluten-containing grains), dairy, processed sugars, soy, and corn. You'll also avoid white potatoes and white rice during the first thirty days. Later I'll show you how to invite some of these back into your life again.

Remember to drink two glasses of filtered or real spring water before each meal, with more throughout the day between meals. I love starting my day with a glass of Sole (pronounced solay) Himalayan salt water for the mineral content (see page 281 for instructions on how to make it). Try it!

Monday:

- Breakfast: 2 pastured eggs, soft poached with spinach sautéed in olive oil and a dash of salt + 2 strips pastured bacon + 1 cup boiled root vegetables (such as sweet potatoes, carrots, or beets) with ghee, a squeeze of lemon, and sea salt
- Lunch: organic roasted chicken or wild fish with a side of leafy greens and vegetables sautéed in ghee and garlic
- Dinner: **Meat Sauce** (page 281) over sweet potatoes + steamed broccoli and asparagus with lemon, salt, and olive oil
- Dessert: whole fruit + a small drizzle of honey

Tuesday:

- Breakfast: **KB Smoothie** (page 282)
- Lunch: grass-fed beef (medium-rare) with fresh garden salad
- Dinner: **Chicken Curry** (page 283) over quinoa and unlimited roasted vegetables
- Dessert: 2 to 3 squares of dark chocolate

Wednesday:

- Breakfast: **Seed Cereal** (page 284) + optional hard-boiled egg dipped in olive oil with a squeeze of lemon and sea salt
- Lunch: Boneless and skinless sardines (unless you want to go for the whole fish!) with a side of sauerkraut or kimchi + avocado with sunflower seeds topped with olive oil, apple cider vinegar, and salt
- Dinner: **Ghee Poached Salmon** (page 284) with **Cauliflower Rice** (page 285) and zucchini sautéed in coconut oil with garlic and cilantro.
- Dessert: **Avocado Chocolate Mousse (**page 285) topped with cinnamon and honey or maple syrup

Thursday:

- <u>Breakfast:</u> **Paleo Pancakes** (page 286) with ghee
- <u>Lunch:</u> Fresh garden salad topped with grilled fish or chicken
- <u>Dinner:</u> Grilled steak and roasted root vegetables
- <u>Dessert:</u> **Coconut Crack Bars** (page 286)

Friday:

- <u>Breakfast:</u> **Zucchini with Ground Beef and Cumin** (page 287)
- <u>Lunch:</u> **Kelly's Chef's Salad** (page 287)
- <u>Dinner:</u> **Rosemary Mustard Lamb Chops** (page 288) with sautéed collard greens and quinoa
- <u>Dessert:</u> **Golden Tea with Coconut Milk** (page 288)

Saturday:

- <u>Breakfast:</u> **KB Smoothie** (page 282)
- <u>Lunch:</u> Prosciutto rolls (arugula tossed in lemon juice and olive oil wrapped in prosciutto)
- <u>Dinner:</u> **Nonna's "Fried" Chicken** (page 289) with **Coconut Cauliflower Rice** (page 285).
- <u>Dessert:</u> **Honey Nut Bars** (page 289)

Sunday:

- <u>Breakfast:</u> 2 pastured eggs, soft poached with spinach sautéed in olive oil and a dash of salt + 2 strips pastured bacon + 1 cup boiled root vegetables (such as sweet potatoes, carrots, and beets)
- <u>Lunch:</u> **Butternut Squash Lasagna Without the Lasagna** (page 290)
- <u>Dinner:</u> **Meatloaf** (page 291) with **Sautéed Red Cabbage and Capers** (page 292)
- <u>Dessert:</u> 2 squares of dark chocolate dipped in 1 tablespoon almond butter

The most important lesson to learn as you embark on this new way of eating (and living!) is to begin to listen to your body. It knows what it wants. When we clear the slate of processed foods designed to bait your animal brain into addiction, we begin to guide ourselves toward our best diet. We've known about our body's inner intelligence anecdotally for centuries, and more scientifically since 1939, when Chicago pediatrician Clara M. Davis presented the stunning results of an experiment that demonstrated body wisdom. Body wisdom is an instinctive attraction to the foods that our body needs for nutrition. It tells us exactly what, when, and how much to eat. We all have this intuition, just as animals in the wild do. Davis proved her point using children, suspecting that children would eat exactly what they needed nutritionally if presented with a cornucopia of healthy foods to choose from. And she was right. Her findings, published in the *Canadian Medical Association Journal,* changed the advice of pediatricians across North America.[1] Emotional or compulsive overeating (eating when you're not hungry to meet emotional needs and cravings) and eating processed foods, which are engineered to disrupt body wisdom so you eat more and more of the wrong food, are what interfere most with body wisdom.

Let's say you feel like a new person after a month of dietary change, but then you eat a bagel—the same bagel you'd been eating for thirty-some-odd years—and you develop a headache and can't remember your password at the bank. You have now defined a linear cause–and–effect relationship in what would otherwise be a sea of dots. This new way of eating is about self-education and mindfulness.

As you go through the program, begin to pay attention to your cravings and preferences. How often do you feel like eating red meat? Two to three times per week or every day? Are you craving fruit, or can you take it or leave it? What about greens? Are you eating them just because they are good for you or because you love them? If you just listen to your body, you will begin to fall into your best diet, the diet that most complements your nervous system and balances your physiology.

> ### MINDFUL EATING
>
> As we participate in the transfer of energy that is the food chain, it is important to cultivate mindfulness around the food we eat. Take one to three breaths with your eyes closed before each meal and express gratitude for the journey that your food took to get to you, to integrate into your being, and to keep you nourished.

WEEK 2: HOME DETOX

In Chapter 8 I gave you lots of ideas for greening your home and environment. During the second week, I encourage you to go back to that chapter and begin to implement a cleanup on the home front. Start with the easy stuff: swapping out toxic cleaning supplies, toiletries, beauty products, and cosmetics for natural alternatives. Plan how you'll update any big-ticket household necessities such as mattresses, furniture, and flooring. And bring in some plants such as Gerbera daisies and English ivy to naturally detoxify the air. Place water filters on your sinks and showerheads.

During this week, aim to try out one or more of the following:

- Dry skin brushing (see page 206)
- Daily coffee enema and two Epson salt baths (see box on page 257)
- Bentonite clay (see below)

    Bentonite, also known as montmorillonite, is composed of aged volcanic ash and is one of the most effective and powerful healing clays. The name comes from the largest known deposit of bentonite clay, located in Fort Benton, Wyoming. Bentonite clay is unique in its ability to produce an electrical charge upon contact with fluid, enabling it to absorb and remove toxins, heavy metals, impurities, and chemicals. Bentonite clay is a common ingredient in detox and cleansing products and can be used externally as a clay poultice or mud pack, in the bath, and in skin care protocols. It has a very fine, velveteen feel and is odorless and non-staining. A good quality bentonite is sourced as a liquid. For internal cleansing, try drinking 1 tablespoon of liquid bentonite in a cup of water most days.

COFFEE ENEMAS

While it may sound unusual, there's nothing new about coffee enemas. Physicians and naturopathic practitioners have used them for a long time to address all sorts of conditions, from constipation and liver detoxification to chronic fatigue, insomnia, and cancer. In fact, when I learned about the power of coffee enemas from Dr. Gonzalez, he showed me a 1932 paper from the *New England Journal of Medicine* that describes resolution of symptoms from depression to psychosis and discharge from inpatient units by simply employing coffee enemas.[2] Coffee delivered to the rectum isn't the same as drinking coffee; the effects are dramatically different. Among the benefits of coffee enemas: when you introduce coffee through the rectum, its compounds stimulate a reflex in the colon that supports liver detox processes as well as bile secretion for improved digestion. This reflex is a parasympathetic one, so the experience is quite different from the sympathetic stimulation of drinking coffee.

Here's how to perform a basic coffee enema:

Brew: Using a French press, brew 2 tablespoons of organic coffee with 1 quart of boiled filtered water for 5 minutes, then press. Let cool in room temperature until it reaches body temperature (2 to 3 hours). Fill the enema container—a 2-quart enema bag and a plastic or stainless-steel bucket with a clamp.

Remove air: Remove any air from the enema tube by grasping but not closing the clamp on the hose. Place the tip in the sink. Hold up the enema bag above the tip until the water begins to flow out. Then close the clamp. This expels any air in the tube.

Lubricate: Lubricate the enema tip with a small amount of coconut oil.

Position yourself: Lie on your left side.

Place the container above you: With the clamp closed, hang the bag about one foot above your abdomen or rest the bucket on a nearby sink.

Insert: Insert the tip gently and slowly about twelve inches in.

Open flow: Open the clamp and hold the enema bag about one foot above the abdomen. The water may take a few seconds to begin flowing. If you develop a cramp, close the hose clamp, turn from side to side, and take a few deep breaths. The cramp usually will pass quickly.

Retain half of the volume for ten minutes, then expel and repeat once.

To watch a video with step-by-step instructions of performing an enema, go to my website, www.kellybroganmd.com.

For a detox period, daily enemas are most effective along with twice-weekly fifteen-minute Epsom soda baths, which you can make by adding 1 cup of baking soda and 1 cup of Epsom salts to your bath.

WEEK 3: PEACE OF MIND

Now that you've been on the protocol for a couple of weeks, you should be feeling a little better. Have your sugar cravings waned? Are you feeling a bit lighter on your feet? Clearer in your mind? Less symptomatic of "depression"?

I've got two goals for you this week. One is to start your core supplements (see below), and two is to engage in a daily meditation practice. Refer back to the strategies in Chapter 7 and find a technique that works for you, whether it's taking three minutes for some deep breathing in the morning and at night or sitting in mindful silence for eleven minutes and summoning feelings of gratitude. Try a kundalini yoga class at a nearby studio sometime this week or get a video to use at home. Schedule these important practices into your life.

Start Your Core Supplements

This week you will be starting a daily supplement regimen. All of the supplements listed below can be found at health food stores, most drugstores and supermarkets, and online. For the record, I do not have any financial relationships with any supplement or device companies. But I am often asked about brands, and I find myself naming certain brands because I know they are good quality and live up to my expectations. I don't want people who are trying to follow my protocol to buy products that are of poor quality or that can even be dangerous if sourced and manufactured poorly. I've included a list of some of my favorite brands at www.kellybroganmd.com. Feel free to purchase other brands so long as you do your homework and know the quality of the ingredients.

For more details about these supplements, refer back to Chapter 9. If you have any questions about personal dosages, ask your doctor for help in making proper adjustments.

▶ B complex (remember to look for a B complex that contains folate as 5-methyltetrahydrofolate and B_{12} as methylcobalamin, hydroxocobalamin, or adenosylcobalamin)
▶ A multimineral that contains magnesium, zinc, iodine, and selenium
▶ A fatty acid that contains EPA and DHA and one with GLA (from evening primrose oil)
▶ Adrenal glandular
▶ Digestive enzymes/pancreatic enzymes

Know How to Get Out of Your Own Way:
Surrender to the Flow

In Chapter 7 I described the influence that Michael Singer's book *The Untethered Soul* had on me. I never would have picked it up if it hadn't been given to me. His beautiful words opened me up in a powerful way. No unicorns and butterflies—this book presents a matter-of-fact option for happiness and freedom. We each have a choice: engage in the process of surrender to the flow or stay in chronic suffering punctuated by acute experiences of victimization and trauma.

In Singer's second work, aptly called *The Surrender Experiment,* he chronicles the mind-expanding experiences that surfaced when he decided to let go; when he decided to just show up to life every day and to stop trying to make it happen the way he thought he wanted it to. Singer writes: "Challenging situations create the force needed to bring about change. The problem is that we generally use all the stirred-up energy intended to bring about change to resist change. I was learning to sit quietly in the midst of the howling winds and wait to see what constructive action was being asked of me."[3]

As a hot-headed Irish-Italian, these words taught me what will be at the core of my personal work for the years to come—watch, observe, and wait for the peak emotion to pass before acting. For many of my patients, this means taking a look at distress, hopelessness, and upset and allowing the feelings to be so the wave of emotions can crest and fall. It means getting acquainted with neutral mind—that nonparticipatory bystander without preferences.

How? In this model, you choose to get out of your own way by allowing the constant chatter of the mind to atrophy—by ignoring that annoying voice that is constantly second-guessing, criticizing, panicking, plotting.

You are not those thoughts. You are the one witnessing those thoughts. All you are here to do is remain open to what is put in your path and in your hands. To accept the flow. To appreciate the unexpected growth that manifests out of adversity. In moments of tension, discomfort, or even agony, try this:

- ▸ Notice and acknowledge your discomfort.
- ▸ Relax and release it no matter how urgent it feels to act.
  Let the energy pass through you before you attempt to fix anything.
- ▸ Imagine sitting up high as you watch your thoughts, emotions, and behavior with a detached compassion.
- ▸ Then ground yourself. Connect to the present moment—feel the earth under your feet, smell the air, imagine roots growing into the earth from your spine.

Practice this strategy this week; it only takes a few minutes. I never expect my patients to diminish the stress in their life. I do, however, expect them to work to shift their perspectives on it—to see and accept their reality so that it can change organically when they stop fighting with it. To continuously let go of attachment to outcome. To work daily on getting the ego out of the way of spirit.

I ask my patients to start with three minutes. Everyone has three minutes. These minutes add up and will make the goals of week 4 effortless.

WEEK 4: MOVEMENT AND SLEEP

Time to get moving if you don't already keep an exercise routine. If you've been sedentary, start with five to ten minutes of burst exercise (thirty seconds of maximal effort and ninety seconds of recovery) and work up to twenty minutes at least three times a week. This can be done any number of ways, such as walking outside and varying your speed and levels of intensity with hills, using classic gym equipment, or watching online videos to perform a routine in the comfort of your home.

For those of you who already maintain a fitness regimen, see if you can increase your workouts to a minimum of thirty minutes a day at least five days a week. This also might be the week you try something different, such as a dance class, dropping in on a yoga studio, or calling a friend who you know is an exercise fiend and asking for help and ideas. These days opportunities to exercise go far beyond traditional gyms, so there's really no excuse. I really don't care which you choose—just pick one! Get out your calendar and schedule your physical activity.

Once you've gotten a regular workout in your schedule, you can include different types of exercise in your daily routine. For some, repetition is key, and for others, variety is important. I like variety and efficiency. I do a short kundalini yoga set daily, a full kundalini class once or twice a week, twenty minutes of burst training on the elliptical once a week, hip-hop dance class once a week, and spinning once or twice a week. That's enough to keep me going strong!

On days when there's absolutely no time to devote to formal exercise, think about ways of sneaking in some physical activity during the day. Research indicates that you can get similar health benefits from three ten-minute bouts of exercise as you would from a single thirty-minute workout. So if you are short on time on any given day, break up your routine into bite-size chunks. And think of how you can combine exercise with other tasks; for example, conduct a meeting with a work colleague while walking outside, or complete a set of stretching exercises while watching television at night. If possible, limit the time you spend sitting down. Walk around while you're on the phone, take the stairs rather than the elevator, and park far away from the entrance to your building. The more you move throughout the day, the more your body—and mood—benefits.

In addition to establishing better exercise habits, use this week to focus on your sleep. If you get less than six hours of sleep a night, start by increasing it to at least seven hours. This is the bare minimum if you want to have normal levels of fluctuating hormones in your body. In addition to the guidance offered in Chapter 7, here are my top three tips for getting a good night's sleep:

Be ritualistic with your sleep habits

Go to bed and get up at roughly the same time daily no matter what. Keep your bedtime routine consistent; it might include downtime, a warm bath, or whatever you need to do to wind down and signal to your body that it's time for sleep. We give our children bedtime rituals but often forget about our own. Rituals work wonders to help us to feel primed for slumber. And don't forget to keep your bedroom quiet, dark, and electronic-free.

Time your last meal smartly

Leave approximately three hours between dinner and bedtime so your stomach is settled and poised for you to go to sleep. Avoid late-night eating. If you need a bedtime snack, try a handful of nuts.

Make sure you're not cheating

You already know that coffee acts as a stimulant, but so can food colorings, flavorings, sugar, and other refined carbs. If you follow my dietary protocol, you're not likely to encounter these. But if you cheat, the consequences might interfere with your sleep.

By the time you reach the end of the first thirty days, you should be in the groove and feeling much better than you did a month ago. Don't panic if you don't feel like you've totally hit your stride yet. Most of us have at least one weak spot in our lives that requires extra attention. Perhaps you're the type who has a hard time saying no to people who will unwittingly attempt to derail you at a party with friends (think booze and inflammatory foods), or maybe finding the time to exercise is exceedingly challenging given your personal demands. Use this fourth week to find a rhythm in your new routine. Identify areas in your life in which you struggle to maintain the protocol and see what you can do to rectify them. Then ask yourself the question *Now what?*

BEYOND THE THIRTY DAYS: BRINGING BACK SOME FOODS AS A BALANCED CARNIVORE

Here's how to reintroduce some of the foods that were sidelined during the first thirty days:

Grains, white rice, white potatoes, and beans

After the thirty days, pick a day to have white potatoes with a meal—boil or steam them and cool them before eating so they are more starch resistant. Eat a big portion and see how you feel. Monitor your system for fatigue, gas, bloating, or brain fog. After three days, try white rice—make sure it's cooled before eating. At this point, most of my patients experience notable improvement in their microbial ecosystem and these resistant starches are well tolerated. For many, beans that are soaked before cooking can also be well tolerated. If they cause gas or bloating, it's not a problem to live without them. When you introduce them, try one type at a time in a significant quantity (2 to 3 servings in a day) and continue to avoid soy (because of antithyroid and antipancreas effects).

Dairy

Many of my patients do not go back to dairy. If you are curious about incorporating it back into your diet, begin with the forms that are least likely to cause problems (see below), eat it at least two times in one day, and watch for three days. Most patients experience fatigue, gas, bloating, or nausea if tolerance is an issue. Introduce dairy in this order:

1. Fermented goat's/sheep's milk dairy
2. Goat's/sheep's milk cheese
3. Grass-fed cow's butter (low in casein)

I typically do not recommend adding back cow's milk cheese or liquid because of how difficult it can be to source A2 beta-casein milk in this country (the type of casein less likely to cause problems) and because of "silent" inflammatory responses, but if you do want to see how you tolerate it, introduce it in this order:

1. Heavy cream
2. Fermented cow's milk dairy
3. Hard cow's milk cheese
4. Cow's milk

Remember that dairy should be raw and grass-fed, which may represent a logistical hurdle for many (see www.rawdairy.com and www.realmilk.com for more information).

Alcohol

I practice in New York City, where drinking alcohol is as much a part of the culture as walking. It is an environment that in many ways is not conducive to the highest vibration of health. That said, learning about your relationship to alcohol is critical. I have many patients who never expected that alcohol was affecting them note that after thirty days it may have been the most important elimination. If you choose to start drinking again after the thirty days, make it an organic wine or a liquor such as gin or tequila with citrus and pay close attention to the effects. What happens to your mood? Your sleep? Does your heart race? Is your brain cloudy two days later? This will help assess its impact so that you can connect cause and effect in the future.

THE BALANCING ACT

As with so many things in life, discovering and establishing a new habit is a balancing act. Even once you've shifted your eating and changed the way you buy, cook, and order food, you'll still have moments when old habits try to emerge. Now that you have the knowledge, I hope that you will stay mindful of your body's true needs every day as best you can. Whenever you feel like you're

METABOLIC TYPE BALANCED CARNIVORE

Meats

POULTRY & FISH 2-3X A WEEK

RED MEAT 3-5X A WEEK
* beef, lamb, and pork, organ meats such as liver, heart, or kidney

RAW MILK/YOGURT: DAILY IF TOLERATED

EGGS 1-2X DAILY

Fruits

BEST
* Bananas, cranberries, plums, and the tropical fruits

MINIMAL FRUITS
* apples, bananas, berries, cantaloupe, cherries, citrus (oranges, grapefruit, lemons, limes, tangerines), coconuts, grapes, kiwi, melons, nectarines, pears, peaches, plums, pomegranates, and tropical fruit such as mango, papaya, and pineapple.

Vegetables

BEST WITH ROOT VEGGIES
* Beets, carrots, potatoes, sweet potatoes, turnips and yams

ACCEPTABLE VEGETABLES
* Spinach (leafy greens <1x a day), asparagus, artichokes, avocado, broccoli, mushroom, nightshade, onion, peas, sea veggies, squash, fermented vegetables

Grains

3-4 TIMES A WEEK
* Rice, Quinoa, Buckwheat, Oats, Millet

Beans

BEST
* aduki beans, black beans, chickpeas (also called garbanzo beans), green beans, kidney beans, lentils, lima beans, navy beans, peas, and pinto beans

Nuts/Seeds

BEST
* Almonds, brazil nuts, cashews, coconuts, filberts, pecans, and walnuts, chia, pine nuts, pistachio, pumpkin, sesame, and sunflower

HONEY, MAPLE SYRUP, MOLASSES OK

50% COOKED

Nicholas Gonzalez, M.D.

about to fall off the proverbial wagon, commit to the same four weeks of the strict protocol again. It can be your lifeline to a healthier way of living that supports the vision you have for yourself. In my experience, even two weeks of recommitting to the slate-clearing template can relieve symptoms aggravated by cheats on vacation or at a dinner party.

You know that life is an endless series of choices. *Eat this or that? Wear this or that? Today or tomorrow? Plan A or B?* The mission of this book is to help you learn to make better decisions that will ultimately allow you to participate in life at its fullest. My hope is that I've given you plenty of ideas to at least begin to make a difference in your life. I see the value that feeling vibrant and healthy brings to people every day in my practice. I also see what chronic disease and depression can do regardless of people's achievements and how much they are loved.

When we sit in stillness and watch, we can see just what is in store for us. Sometimes challenges are exactly what the doctor ordered. Sometimes tragedy is part of our path; other times, something amazing can turn out to be a colossal burden. In the world of psychiatry, distress is a sign of sickness to be eliminated by consciousness-suppressing drugs instead of a gateway to change, an invitation to look at and fix what might be misaligned or out of balance. Whatever has brought you to this book is something to be grateful for. It's what you needed to raise your awareness and to ready yourself to pass over a threshold. May my message and ideas be a gateway to change.

SPECIAL CIRCUMSTANCES: TAPERING FROM MEDS AFTER THE THIRTY DAYS

Eva had been taking an antidepressant for two years, but now wanted to get off it because she was planning to get pregnant. Based on available evidence, her doctor advised her to continue the drug, which motivated her to see me. Eva explained that her saga had begun with

PMS, featuring a week each month when she was irritable and prone to crying fits. Her doctor prescribed birth control pills (a common treatment), and soon Eva was feeling even worse, with insomnia, fatigue, low libido, and a generally flat mood dogging her all month long. That's when the doctor added Wellbutrin to "pick her up," as he put it, and handle her presumed depression. From Eva's perspective, she felt that the antidepressant helped her energy level but had limited benefits in terms of her mood and irritability. And if she took it after midnight, her insomnia was exacerbated. She soon became accustomed to feeling stable but suboptimal, and she was convinced that the medication was keeping her afloat.

The good news for Eva was that with careful preparation she could leave medication behind—and restore her energy, her equilibrium, and her sense of control over her emotions. Step one was my thirty-day program. Step two involved stopping birth control pills and testing her hormone levels. Just before her period, she had low cortisol and progesterone, which were likely the cause of the PMS that started her whole problem. Further testing revealed borderline low thyroid function, which may well have been the result of the contraceptives—and the cause of her increased depressive symptoms.

When Eva was ready to begin tapering off her medication, she did so following my protocol. Even as her brain and body adjusted to no longer having the SSRI surging through her system, her energy levels improved, her sleep problems resolved, and her anxiety lifted. Within a year she was healthy, no longer taking any prescriptions, with normalized thyroid function, feeling good—and pregnant.

Judging by the most heavily trafficked articles on my website and my practice's FAQ, this will be the most important section of the book for many people. It is not easy to get off psychiatric medications once you start. It's not even easy to get information on how to wean yourself safely from them. You'll hear "talk to your doctor before discontinuing" and get advice to taper off gradually, and these are reasonable first steps. But this is not nearly enough information to allow you to stop successfully.

No one is more vested in safely and effectively discontinuing psych meds than pregnant women—or, more specifically, women planning to get pregnant. This is a specialty of mine in my practice. Pregnant or planning-to-be-pregnant women don't need anything more or less than the next person in the waiting room does. The way you prepare your body to come off medication without ill effect is, in many respects, the same as how you'd prepare your body for pregnancy. In both cases, optimal results come from being in the best possible shape before embarking on this new journey. I'll be honest: some people who currently are taking antidepressants won't be able to safely taper and may have to continue using the drugs indefinitely or until medicine has better solutions. Still, what I've shared in this book will help you find more relief and you'll fare better than if you were solely depending on antidepressants without making any other changes.

What has fueled my fire about the irresponsible prescribing of psychiatric medications is bearing witness to cases of severe discontinuation syndrome. This refers to the months to years of nervous system instability that can result from medication taper. The process of coming off of antidepressants is just that, a process. If you've been treated for longer than two months, the process must be slow with small incremental decreases in medication doses and use of liquid preparations and compounds when small increments are not available. Of course this will require the help of a physician—one who supports your willingness to taper and to do so in a responsible, safe manner. The reason you must invest in those first thirty days of dietary change is to promote resilience before tapering off so that your body will be able to adapt to the change. It's the idea of draining your bucket so that it doesn't overflow when the "Where-are-my-meds?!" brain and body bomb drops.

Each person's experience in the tapering off process will be different. Sadly, I was taught to dismiss patients concerned about becoming "addicted" to psych meds and to deny the possibility of protracted withdrawal, describing it only as evidence of that patient's clear "need" for permanent medication treatment.

I was never taught how to taper. In the first systematized review of SSRI withdrawal, researchers examined twenty-three studies and thirty-eight case reports, leading them to conclude that the euphemistic term *discontinuation syndrome* must be abandoned in lieu of a more accurate depiction of the habit-forming qualities of antidepressants: withdrawal. Yes, just like Xanax, Valium, alcohol, and heroin. In the words of McGill University's Chouinard and Chouinard, two researchers in the Departments of Psychiatry and Medicine: "[P]atients can experience classic new withdrawal symptoms, rebound and/or persistent postwithdrawal disorders, or relapse/recurrence of the original illness. New and rebound symptoms can occur for up to six weeks after drug withdrawal, depending on the drug elimination half-life, while persistent postwithdrawal or tardive disorders associated with longlasting receptor changes may persist for more than six weeks after drug discontinuation."[4]

They provide a handy chart of the horrors that can befall unsuspecting patients, ranging from those who miss a dosage to those who taper carefully. A rare instance of clinical documentation on tapering patients is offered by Dr. Jonathan Prousky; in one of his seminal papers, he describes in detail his approach to complex cases. He supports the patient's reframing of their experience of mental illness, their self-care, and a careful dosage schedule that involves decreasing medication and use of natural agents such as nicotinamide (B_3), botanicals such as rhodiola rosea, and amino acids such as GABA and L-theanine. He concurs, as do I, that there is no magic supplement bullet, and that the most important thing to do is to use dietary strategies and supplements known for their antidepression effects and promotion of the relaxation of the nervous system. After all, these effects are the ultimate goal.

Giving each reader her unique tapering protocol is beyond the scope of this book. But if you've taken my ideas to heart and have successfully completed the thirty days, then you've already given yourself the best head start to finding your exit door, and you are ready to start that process with a supportive doctor who can tailor your treatment.

The treatment team partnership is critical, with the most op-timal results coming from lifestyle change, careful management of dosage decreases, and strategic support through nutraceuticals. Most patients and their practitioners know that the dosages made available by pharmaceutical companies are not conducive to a suc-cessful taper. Liquid preparations, compounding pharmacies, and even meticulous removal of beads from capsules are indispensable work-around tools you can talk about with your doctor.

Keep in mind that the risk of relapse is often related to the nature of the effects the medication has on the brain and body. In my ex-perience, agitation, anxiety, and insomnia are the most common symptoms of withdrawal, and they can crop up within hours of a dose change or sometimes several months after the final dose. They can resolve spontaneously, or they can come back. Long-term damage from these medications is a real phenomenon, and one that is poorly understood outside of patient accounts and peer support groups. But patients are rarely wrong.

You're not alone if you're taking an antidepressant, even though you might *feel* alone in so many ways. Millions of people find them-selves caught in the web of psychiatric sorcery—a spell potentially cast for life. Like you, they are told that they have chemical imbal-ances. They are told that the most important thing they can do for themselves is to "take their medication," and that they will have to do so "for life." As Dr. Joanna Moncrieff states: "Symbolically, medication suggests that the problem is within the brain and well-being is dependent upon maintaining 'chemical balance' by artifi-cial means. This message encourages patients to view themselves as flawed and vulnerable and may explain the poor outcomes of treated depression in naturalistic studies."

These patients have suffered a crisis of resiliency.

The stress of their life experience outpaced what their physical resources could support. Providers are not asking *why* they became sick when they did. They are not exploring root causes. I realize I'm probably sounding like a broken record at this point, but now that we've come full circle, it's important that I drive this point home again. If you're taking an antidepressant, then chances are your doctor is not discussing evidence-based alternatives to medication treatment. And he or she is not disclosing the long-term risks of psychotropics including worse results and increased risk of relapse—let alone the poor integrity and industry-funded and manipulated data that supports the approval for efficacy of these medications.

Most egregiously, you're being sold the belief that medication is treating your disease rather than inducing a drug effect no different from alcohol or cocaine. If a single dose of an antidepressant can change the architecture of the brain in ways we have no science to appreciate, what are the results of chronic, long-term use? What happens when patients want out? When they are not happy with treatment? When they make sufficient changes in their lives to support a new approach?

As psychiatrist and activist Peter Breggin has stated, medication withdrawal programs are the most urgently needed intervention in the field of psychiatry.[5]

I have few like-minded colleagues. Most of what I have learned about psychiatric drug withdrawal I have learned from patients and from clinical experience. The best way to promote resiliency is to bring back a signal of safety to the mind and body. And that signal comes in the form of simple lifestyle habits via nutrition, a clean environment, an ideal light cycle throughout the day and night, as well as movement; the evidence for these strategies is amassing in the literature.

In addition to the basic how-tos I've described in this book, one of the most important steps is to change your mind. You need to change your mind to have a mind of your own. In other words, don't be afraid. This is what I counsel patients on the most. Fear is the enemy of health. Fear is what brings people to psychiatrists, pushes 911 on the phone, and drives an urgent feeling of hopeless overwhelm. Psychiatrists are driven by fear and a need to control and regulate the emotional experience. As healers, we have the opportunity to meet this fear with compassion and equanimity. We can put aside our obsessive preoccupation with reactive intervention and liability-driven care and learn to tolerate what is uncomfortable about a patient's distress. Given that the data supports the undeniable fact that the current model of medication-based intervention is failing, we must do this.

Once you've completed the first thirty days to a T, there is a strong possibility that the original driver of your symptoms has been addressed. You may not have the same need for your medication or be deriving much benefit from it. I believe it is each person's choice to manage their health in a way that resonates with their beliefs about health and wellness. This decision should be made with eyes wide open and preferably with gentle interventions preceding more aggressive ones. The complexity of the body is awe-inspiring, and depression is a syndrome that has many different causes. Look to the root, look to healing, and look to restoration for real lasting change. Use the tools I've given you and come back to this book whenever you need reminders. Employ the power of the Internet as well: visit my website for more updated material and go to places like the support forums on www.madinamerica.com to connect with others and access a variety of resources.

I believe in transferring a sense of empowerment to my patients. I talk to them about this process as being one of rebirth—of a rising from the ash—and a deliberate step in the direction of wholeness and radiant life.

Because health—and life—is so much more than the absence of pills and the fading of a laundry list of diagnoses. Health is liberation. And it's a basic human right.

Own Your Body and Free Your Mind

In fact, I am certain, there has never been a
doctor anywhere, at any time, in any country,
at any period in history who ever healed anything.
Each person's healer is within.
—MARLO MORGAN, *MUTANT MESSAGE DOWN UNDER*

Before you close this book, let me share with you a little something I learned recently that has made a difference in my life. In the end I didn't write this book just to offer my take on the new psychiatry. It's also about the new feminism. Here's what I mean by that.

When my beloved teacher and kundalini guide, Swaranpal Kaur Khalsa, told me about the symbology of *Adi Shakti,* one of the most ancient symbols of the sacred feminine, I knew *this* was where I needed to take my patients. *Adi Shakti* is made up of four symbolic weapons that represent primal creative feminine power from a tradition that champions all that is incomparable about a woman's energy.

In this depiction, every female is charged with balancing the woman and the mother:

"As a mother you are supposed to sacrifice, tolerate, be very patient, be very thoughtful of others, and understand all the pros and cons of any situation. As a woman you must give nothing; you have to protect yourself first; and you need not tolerate any nonsense. Woman must be able to ascertain which is the correct relationship—woman or mother," sword or shield.[1]

The sword is her incisive determination to dedicate herself to a path of truth, intolerance of assault, and fierce rejection of all that comes between her intuition and her integrity. As she is a warrior, she is also a nurturer.

It has been my mission to help women reclaim that inner compass, pick up their swords, and defend the enigma of their most unquantifiable beauty and power. It is my grave concern that this power has been co-opted by a paternalistic system that seeks to engender fear and control by coercion and undermine a woman's inner voice by suggesting that science has cracked the code of the human condition. A system that turns a blind eye to all the times science and medicine have been in error. That we as a society have let fear lead us down a shameful path.

Many of you will feel you don't have the space or energy to pick up this sword, to recapture the true meaning of health, peace, and happiness. I argue that you don't have the space or energy *not* to. If you've gotten to this point in the book, I trust you're ready. And you know now that you must make the space and time to move forward with resolve.

In today's health climate, a failure to challenge industry, government, and media claims can lead you and your family down a lonely road of remorse, heartache, and financial ruin. As Elizabeth Lesser, author of *Broken Open,* says, every experience of struggle offers us what we need to be born anew. These are ways that we achieve enlightenment and a connection to our primal power. We are told that feelings of discomfort are nuisances to be medicated away. We are herded like cattle into holding pens of conformity.

I am here to tell you that saying yes to yourself begins with saying no to the medical-agricultural-industrial complex, and to help inspire those of you open enough to feel it, to begin to *wonder*. To begin to experience gratitude for what is. I like to call this a position of personal nonresistance. While we hold our swords aloft, we simultaneously access a softness, a yielding, an acceptance for what happens here on the ground. This is balancing the woman with the mother. It's fighting so that we can love better, freer, with less fear. This is living mindfully in a state of calm alertness.

Begin to tap into all that is beyond the grasp of allopathic medicine. Take it back and rise up with a new kind of feminism—one with women banding together, talking to one another, trusting in their guts, and building a model of health that is so compelling that the current model will soon be revealed for its transparent agenda, missteps, and offenses. This is where your power lies. Once you taste it, the world will know, and there will be no stopping you.

THE RELIGION OF MEDICINE[2]

I used to think that religious dogma was the outgrowth of fear and unresolved parental issues. Certainly, much modern religion has lost touch with its more mystical roots, but there is no question that what ails the average American, as British writer and journalist Graham Hancock says, is a disconnection from Spirit.

When we disconnect from a sense of inner guidance and intuition, we are forced to rely on external constructs, on blind faith in authority, and so-called experts. The truth is that you are your own best authority, but you have to get excited about your new position. You must trust to have faith that it will unfold in your best interest if you just relax into the process. My mentor Dr. Nicholas Gonzalez said, "Patients have to do the treatment they believe in. Fear is an infectious disease. You can catch fear but you can't catch faith. That has to come from within."

I have always practiced this ethos. I know that fear has a nocebo (literally "shall cause harm") effect, the negative effect from a belief that something will harm, that cannot be undone. It's the opposite of the placebo effect.

But where there is faith in the body's ability to heal when properly supported, magical things can happen.

Once we have fed ourselves and put a roof over our heads, then we can concern ourselves with external dangers, then with relationships, then with self-love, then with spirituality and coming in touch with our own power. This is classically known as Maslow's hierarchy, from the famous psychologist's paper on the subject in 1943 called "A Theory of Human Motivation."[3]

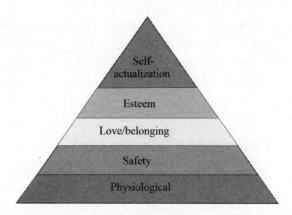

Of course, many of us can get stuck today pinballing between the lower three rungs on the ladder, never quite making it to the apical agenda. I see the work of teaching patients about lifestyle medicine as having the unintended benefit of radically changing, evolving, and freeing one's life path to discover purpose-driven behaviors.

We all want to know and connect to our purpose in this life. We want to know what we are here for. But how can we bother with that if we are plagued by fears of degenerative conditions and chronic ill health and bogged down under labels and diagnoses?

When the body comes into harmony, it's more than just symptom relief; it's an opportunity to come into yourself and ascend that ladder.

For me I had to heal my body and resolve my autoimmune condition before I could open myself up to my greater mission and to the gifts of a kundalini yoga practice and connection to the power of energy medicine. I understand now that cultivating an inner compass is trusting in a guide inside and connecting without fear to a trust in the unfolding of the universe. An unfolding we are here only to witness. In this way, challenges and distress are an invitation to look at what might be misaligned or out of balance. It's a whole new take on the complexity of life as a woman today.

My hope is that I've given you the tools to find your path.

Own your body. Free your mind. It's so much more than a "cure."

Recipes

The following recipes are arranged in order of mention in the one-week plan. As long as you stick with the main guidelines, you can feel free to have fun with the recipes and make substitutions to cater to your needs and preferences.

SOLE HIMALAYAN SALT WATER

Fill a 16-ounce glass jar a quarter of the way with Himalayan salt or unprocessed sea salt and fill with filtered water. Cover and let sit overnight. Take 1 teaspoon of the mixture and mix it into a glass of filtered water. Drink first thing in the morning. Sole "kits" can also be found online with salt rocks and jars.

MEAT SAUCE

Serves 4 to 6
1 bunch kale, stems removed and leaves torn
Leaves from 1 bunch fresh cilantro
1 onion, chopped
3 beets, scrubbed and chopped
4 carrots, chopped
4 celery sticks, chopped
2 tablespoons grass-fed ghee
1 pound organic grass-fed ground bison or beef
One 24-ounce glass bottle organic crushed tomatoes

1 tablespoon ground turmeric
Unprocessed sea salt and freshly ground black pepper

Combine the kale, cilantro, onion, beets, carrots, and celery in a food processor and pulse until finely chopped but not pureed.

Melt the ghee in a large skillet over medium heat. Add the vegetables and sauté until the onion is translucent, about 3 minutes. Add the bison and cook, stirring and breaking it apart with the spoon, until browned, 3 to 5 minutes. Add the crushed tomatoes and turmeric and season with salt and pepper. Bring to a simmer and simmer for 20 to 30 minutes to allow flavors to combine. Serve over squash, quinoa, or broccoli.

THE KB SMOOTHIE

Serves 1
½ cup frozen organic cherries or other berries
8 ounces coconut water, or filtered water
3 tablespoons collagen hydrolysate (as a protein base; see note following recipe)
1 tablespoon sprouted nut butter or sunflower seed butter
3 large pastured egg yolks
1 tablespoon virgin coconut oil
1 to 2 tablespoons grass-fed ghee
1 to 2 tablespoons raw cocoa powder

Combine all the ingredients in a blender and blend until smooth.

Note: collagen hydrolysate is a protein food supplement high in the amino acids glycine, proline, and lycine. It comes as a dry powder.

CHICKEN CURRY

Serves 4

2 tablespoons coconut oil or ghee

1½ pounds chicken thighs, boneless and skinless, cut into 1-inch pieces

1 medium onion, cut into large chunks

2 zucchini, thickly sliced

1 tablespoon curry powder

½ teaspoon paprika

3 cloves garlic, minced

1 teaspoon unprocessed sea salt

14 ounces unsweetened organic coconut milk (not from a can)

1 cup organic grape tomatoes

¼ cup cilantro, chopped, for garnish

In a stockpot, heat the oil or ghee to medium-high heat, then add chicken and cook until pieces are browned on both sides, 8 to 10 minutes. Remove the chicken from the pan and set aside, leaving the remaining oil in the pot. Add the onion and zucchini and sauté until lightly browned, about 5 minutes. Then add the curry powder, paprika, garlic, and salt and sauté for half a minute. Bring the chicken back to the pot and add coconut milk. Bring to a boil, then reduce heat to a simmer and cover. Cook until chicken is tender, approximately 30 minutes. Add the tomatoes in the final 5 minutes of cooking. Garnish with cilantro.

SEED CEREAL

Serves 1

¼ cup raw nuts and/or seeds of your choice (such as walnuts, pecans, slivered almonds, and pumpkin seeds)

1 tablespoon chia seeds

1 tablespoon flax seeds

1 tablespoon hemp seeds (optional)

½ to 1 cup whole berries or chopped fruit of choice (such as berries, bananas, and nectarines)

1 cup unsweetened almond milk

Combine the nuts and seeds in a bowl. Add the fruit, pour in the almond milk, and serve.

GHEE POACHED SALMON

Serves 2

Two 6-ounce wild Atlantic salmon fillets

1 lemon

4 cloves garlic, crushed

Unprocessed sea salt and freshly ground black pepper

¼ cup grass-fed ghee

¼ cup finely chopped fresh parsley or dill

Place the salmon in a sauté pan with a lid. Squeeze the juice from the lemon over the top, add the garlic, and season with salt and pepper. Slice the remaining spent lemon and spread the slices over the top. Cover and refrigerate for at least 1 hour.

Add the ghee to the pan with the fish. Cover, place over medium heat, and steam until the salmon turns pale orange and is soft in the center. Serve topped with parsley.

CAULIFLOWER RICE

Serves 6
1 large head cauliflower
1 tablespoon extra-virgin olive oil
Unprocessed sea salt

Cut the cauliflower into large pieces, then drop the pieces into the opening in the lid of a food processor until it's three-quarters full (do this in batches if necessary). Pulse until completely broken down into bits the size of couscous.

In a large skillet, heat the oil over medium heat. Add the cauliflower and season with salt, if using. Cover and cook for about 7 minutes, until tender. For a coconut cauliflower rice variation, use coconut oil instead of olive oil and sprinkle with raw shredded coconut at the end.

CHOCOLATE AVOCADO MOUSSE

Serves 4
2 ripe Haas avocados
2 to 4 tablespoons honey or pure maple syrup
⅓ cup raw cacao powder
2 tablespoons unsweetened almond, coconut, or cashew milk
½ teaspoon pure vanilla extract

Scoop the flesh of the avocados into a food processor. Add the honey, cacao powder, almond milk, and vanilla and process until smooth, about 1 minute. Taste and adjust the sweetness with more honey if necessary. Spoon into individual serving dishes, cover, and refrigerate for at least 30 minutes before serving.

PALEO PANCAKES

Serves 1
½ cup cooked sweet potato or winter squash (such as butternut, acorn, or kabocha), or 1 banana
3 large pastured eggs
2 tablespoons hemp seeds, flax seeds, or nut butter
Virgin coconut oil

Combine all the ingredients in a blender and blend until smooth. Spoon silver-dollar-size dollops into medium heat coconut oil. They cook quickly!

COCONUT CRACK BARS

Makes 6 to 8 bars
1 cup unsweetened shredded organic coconut
¼ cup pure maple syrup
2 tablespoons virgin coconut oil
½ teaspoon pure vanilla extract
⅛ teaspoon sea salt
¼ cup dark chocolate chips (optional)

Combine all the ingredients except the chocolate chips in a food processor and pulse to combine well or mix vigorously by hand. Stir in the chocolate chips, if using. Spread firmly into a 7 x 5-inch glass dish and place in the refrigerator for 1 hour or in the freezer for 15 minutes. Cut into 6 to 8 squares. Sprinkle with chocolate chips (optional).

ZUCCHINI WITH GROUND BEEF AND CUMIN

Serves 2 to 3
2 tablespoons grass-fed ghee
½ yellow onion, diced
2 large or 4 small zucchinis, sliced
Dash of unprocessed sea salt
Pinch of ground cumin
Splash of apple cider vinegar
½ pound organic grass-fed ground beef

Heat the ghee in a large sauté pan over medium heat. Add the onion and zucchini and sauté for 5 to 7 minutes, until softened. Stir in the salt, cumin, and vinegar. Add the ground beef and cook, stirring to break it up, for 3 to 5 minutes until browned.

KELLY'S CHEF'S SALAD

Serves 1
One 4 to 5-ounce bag prewashed organic spring lettuce greens
2 hard-boiled eggs, cut in half
½ to 1 cooked organic pastured chicken breast, cut into chunks
2 slices cooked pastured bacon, crumbled
1 large vine-ripened tomato, chopped
½ avocado, cut into chunks
3 green onions, diced
2 celery stalks, diced
½ can anchovies (optional)
Extra-virgin olive oil
Apple cider vinegar
Unprocessed sea salt and freshly ground pepper

Combine the greens, hard-boiled eggs, chicken, bacon, tomato, avocado, green onions, celery, and anchovies, if using, in a salad bowl. Drizzle with olive oil and vinegar and season with salt and pepper.

ROSEMARY MUSTARD LAMB CHOPS

Serves 4

2 tablespoons Dijon-style mustard
2 cloves garlic, minced
2 tablespoons chopped fresh rosemary
8 pinches of unprocessed sea salt and freshly ground black
    pepper
8 organic grass-fed lamb loin chops
1 tablespoon grass-fed ghee

Combine the mustard, garlic, rosemary, salt, and pepper in a small bowl. Rub the mixture evenly over both sides of the lamb chops and place the chops on a baking sheet. Cover and refrigerate for at least 30 minutes.

Melt the ghee in a grill pan over high heat. Add the chops and cook for about 8 minutes on each side, until done to your liking.

GOLDEN TEA WITH COCONUT MILK

Serves 1

1 cup coconut milk
½ teaspoon ground turmeric
1 (½-inch-wide) slice fresh gingerroot, peeled and finely chopped
½ teaspoon ground cinnamon
½ teaspoon raw honey or maple syrup, or to taste
Dash of cayenne pepper (optional)

Combine all the ingredients in a high-speed blender and blend until smooth.

Pour the mixture into a small saucepan and heat over medium heat until hot but not boiling, 3 to 5 minutes. Drink immediately.

NONNA'S "FRIED" CHICKEN

Serves 4

2 tablespoons ghee or extra-virgin olive oil

1 onion, sliced

Unprocessed sea salt and freshly ground black pepper

One 24-ounce jar crushed organic tomato sauce

1 tablespoon virgin coconut oil

1 cup almond flour

2 eggs

1 pound organic pastured chicken cutlets

Melt 1 tablespoon of the ghee in a large sauté pan over medium heat. Add the onion and sauté until softened, about 5 minutes. Season with salt and pepper and add the tomato sauce.

Heat the coconut oil along with the remaining 1 tablespoon ghee in a large skillet over medium heat. Place the almond flour into a shallow bowl and season lightly with salt and pepper. Beat the eggs in a separate shallow bowl. Dip each cutlet into the almond flour, then the eggs, then into the pan with the coconut oil. Cook until golden on each side, 3 to 4 minutes. Move the cutlets into the pan with the tomato sauce, cook for a minute or two to combine, then serve.

HONEY NUT BARS

Serves 12

1 cup cashews

½ cup almonds

½ cup pecans

½ cup unsweetened shredded coconut

½ cup cacao nibs

1 teaspoon pure vanilla extract

½ teaspoon sea salt

9 tablespoons raw honey (a little more than ½ cup)

Preheat the oven to 350°F and line an 8 x 8-inch baking pan with parchment paper.

By hand or using a food processor, roughly chop the nuts into approximately ¼-inch pieces.

Combine all the ingredients except the honey in a large bowl and stir until combined. Add the honey and mix with a fork until the ingredients are evenly coated. Spread the mixture into the pan, pressing down to pack it in and reach all the edges and corners.

Bake for 20 minutes, then cool completely on a wire rack. Lift the whole thing out by the parchment paper and cut into 12 squares.

BUTTERNUT SQUASH LASAGNA WITHOUT THE LASAGNA

Serves 6
1 tablespoon ghee
1 onion, finely diced
1 pound organic grass-fed ground beef or pork
3 garlic cloves, minced
36 ounces organic tomato puree (preferably from a glass jar)
4 ounces organic tomato paste (preferably from a glass jar)
Sea salt and freshly ground black pepper
2 medium or 1 large butternut squash
4 eggs, beaten

Preheat the oven to 400°F.

Melt the ghee in a large sauté pan over medium heat. Add the onion and sauté until softened, about 5 minutes. Add the beef and garlic, raise the heat to medium-high, and cook, breaking the meat apart with a wooden spoon, until the meat is browned, 3 to 5 minutes. Add the tomato puree and tomato paste and season with salt and pepper. Reduce the heat to low and simmer while you prepare the squash.

Peel the squash and slice it into very thin, uniform rounds;

remove the seeds and fiber. Add enough sauce to cover the bottom of a 15 x 10-inch ovenproof dish. Add some squash in a single layer, then add a generous layer of sauce. Add about one-third of the egg and spread it around the dish. Repeat the squash-sauce-egg sequence layering one or two more times depending on how much you have left, finishing with a light layer of sauce.

Bake for 25 to 30 minutes, until a knife easily pierces the squash.

MEATLOAF

Serves 6

1 pound organic grass-fed ground beef
1 pound organic grass-fed ground pork
1 large pastured egg
½ cup organic tomato sauce
1 shallot, finely diced
⅓ cup almond flour
¼ cup diced red bell pepper
1 teaspoon sea salt
½ teaspoon ground celery seed
2 to 3 cloves garlic, minced
Pinch of freshly ground black pepper
2 tablespoons chopped fresh basil (optional)
½ teaspoon smoked paprika (optional)
1 tablespoon organic tomato paste
1 tablespoon yellow mustard

Preheat the oven to 350°F and grease an 8½ x 11-inch baking dish or a loaf pan with ghee.

With clean hands, mix all the meatloaf ingredients (leave the tomato paste and mustard for the sauce) and form into a loaf on the baking dish or into the loaf pan.

Mix the tomato paste and mustard in a small bowl. Brush the sauce over the top of the meatloaf. Bake uncovered for 45 to 60 minutes, until the internal temperature reaches between 175 to 185°F. Remove from the oven and let rest for 15 minutes, then slice and serve with sautéed red cabbage and capers (recipe follows) alongside.

SAUTÉED RED CABBAGE AND CAPERS

Serves 6
2 teaspoons extra-virgin olive oil
1 clove garlic, minced or crushed
1 tablespoon capers
3 ounces red cabbage, chopped
Juice of 1 lemon wedge
Freshly ground black pepper

Heat the oil in a medium skillet over medium heat. Add the garlic and capers and cook for 1 minute. Add the cabbage and sauté for another minute. Squeeze in the lemon juice and cook until the cabbage starts to brown on the edges slightly, 2 to 4 minutes.

BONUS RECIPE: CHICKEN STOCK (MAKE A POT WEEKLY)

1 large onion, coarsely chopped
2 large carrots, chopped
3 celery stalks, chopped
1 (5- to 8-pound) organic pastured chicken, rinsed
2 to 4 tablespoons apple cider vinegar (½ tablespoon per quart of water)
Unprocessed sea salt and freshly ground black pepper
1 bunch (or 10 sprigs) cilantro or parsley, chopped
½ pound chicken livers (optional; when they're finely chopped, you won't taste them and they provide lots of nutrients

Combine all the ingredients in a large stainless-steel stockpot and add cold filtered water to cover. Bring to a boil, then reduce the heat to very low, cover, and simmer for about 3 hours. A pressure cooker will cut the time in half. After the chicken is cooked, the meat can be separated from the bone and used in a shredded-chicken dish by just sautéing the shredded chicken in olive oil and adding salt and lemon.

Acknowledgments

I can only hope to touch the lives of those I am destined to touch and for the doors to be opened to accomplish this. My experience of awakening to the truth has certainly involved struggle, alienation, and loss. Through all of it I have come into contact with my intuition, my innate passion for natural medicine, and my purpose in this life. My path is paved by the minds, hearts, and souls of these people, and for their love I am eternally grateful:

Leela Hatfield, for being my partner in the trenches and my sister everywhere else.

Ron Brogan, for your unwavering devotion and for passing on the gifts of gab, punctuality, and follow-through.

Marusca Brogan, for seeding my soil with feminine empowerment, for predicting this book from my childhood, and for modeling compassion.

Andy Fink, for making this possible, for seeing me, for growing with me, for offering the counsel I seek, and for the most radiant heart I've ever known.

John and Sharkey Fink, for waiting for me to wake up and for showing me how much fun it can be to live in the Truth.

Brendan Brogan, Sara Ojjeh, and Lily and John Harrington, for accepting the challenge of this one wild life with me.

Dean Raffelock, Kat Toups, Michael Schachter, Sylvia Fogel, Alan Logan, and Cornelia Tucker Mazzan, for your generosity, support, and heart-centered companionship on the road toward intellectual freedom.

Joseph Aldo, Olivier Bros, and Laura Kamm, for showing me that energy is the medicine of the future.

James Maskell, for believing that my message belongs in the Evolution of Medicine and health freedom for all.

Kristin Loberg, for giving me an uncensored voice so that I could reach further than I thought possible, for your superlative skills, and for bringing the world's best attitude to my mountains of references, articles, and opinions.

Karen Rinaldi, for your fire, your fearlessness, and for being so refreshingly real (and fun).

Bonnie Solow, for shining your light on me like a ray from on high, and for the incredible pleasure of your charisma, your strength, and your softness.

Lea Pica, for your artistry in shaping my message.

Keith Rhys and Jon Humberstone, for always being right about how to effect change on a global scale.

Omri Chaimovitz, Whitney Burrell, Bipin Subedi, Healy Smith, and Jason Pinto, for showing me unconditional love throughout my Phoenix Process.

Nick Gonzalez, for the treasure of your existence on this human plane and beyond, for showing me the Truth, and how to love it.

Sarah Kamrath, for bringing me to kundalini and for holding this space with me with unparalleled grace.

Sayer Ji, for cracking open my cosmic egg, for our twinship from the academic to the esoteric, and for your vital eye on this manuscript.

Tahra Collins, for your gifts, for loving me, for inspiring me, for traveling this path by my side.

Swaranpal Kaur Khalsa, for being the enlightened midwife of my rebirth.

Louise Kuo Habakus, for our sisterhood of two, for meeting me in the space of fierce righteousness and allowing me to put down my sword long enough to tap into my feminine wisdom.

Sofia and Lucia, for my birth through yours.

My patients, for being my gurus and teaching me what true healing is all about.

The Universe, for the richness of a purpose-driven life.

Notes

INTRODUCTION: PSYCH—IT'S NOT ALL IN YOUR HEAD

1. Troy Brown, "100 Best-Selling, Most Prescribed Branded Drugs Through March [2015]," *Medscape Medical News*, May 6, 2015, www.medscape. com/viewarticle/844317, accessed September 21, 2015.

2. Roni Caryn Rabin, "A Glut of Antidepressants," *New York Times*, August 12, 2013, http://well.blogs.nytimes.com/2013/08/12/a-glut-of-antidepressants/, accessed September 21, 2015.

CHAPTER 1: DECODING DEPRESSION

1. Katherine Bindley, "Women and Prescription Drugs: One in Four Takes Mental Health Meds," *Huffington Post*, November 16, 2011, www.huffingtonpost.com/2011/11/16/women-and-prescription-drug-use_n_1098023.html, accessed September 21, 2015.

2. James Warren, "When Health Care Kills," *New York Daily News*, July 20, 2014, www.nydailynews.com/opinion/health-care-kills-article-1.1872544, accessed September 21, 2015. Also see: J. T. James, "A New, Evidence-based Estimate of Patient Harms Associated with Hospital Care," *J Patient Saf* 9, no. 3 (September 2013): 122–8, doi: 10.1097/ PTS.0b013e3182948a69. This latest study reveals that the Institute of Medicine estimates that up to 98,000 Americans die each year from medical errors alone.

3. "The Third Leading Cause of Death after Heart Disease and Cancer? Experts Debate the Harmful Effects of Psychiatric Medications," Council for Evidence-Based Psychiatry, May 13, 2015, http://cepuk. org/2015/05/13/third-leading-cause-death-heart-disease-cancer-experts-debate-harmful-effects-psychiatric-medications/, accessed September 21, 2015.

4. "Psychiatry Gone Astray," post by Dr. David Healy, January 21, 2014, http://davidhealy.org/psychiatry-gone-astray/, accessed September 21, 2015. Also see: Peter Gøtzsche, *Deadly Medicines and Organised Crime: How*

Big Pharma Has Corrupted Healthcare (New York: Radcliffe Publishing, 2013). For more about Dr. Gøtzsche and his work, go to www. deadlymedicines.dk. And for more about the Cochrane Report, go to www.cochrane.org.

5.   Fiona Godlee, "Balancing Benefits and Harms," *British Medical Journal* 346 (2013): f3666.

6.   V. Prasad et al., "A Decade of Reversal: An Analysis of 146 Contradicted Medical Practices, *Mayo Clinic Proceedings* 88, no. 8 (August 2013): 790–8, doi: 10.1016/j.mayocp.2013.05.012. Epub 2013 Jul 18.

7.   Z. S. Morris, S. Wooding, and J. Grant, "The Answer Is 17 Years, What Is the Question: Understanding Time Lags in Translational Research," *Journal of the Royal Society of Medicine* 104, no. 12 (December 2011): 510–20, doi:10.1258/jrsm.2011.110180.

8.   Richard Horton, "Offline: What Is Medicine's 5 Sigma?" *Lancet* 385 (April 2015).

9.   J. S. Garrow, "What to Do about CAM: How Much of Orthodox Medicine Is Evidence Based?," *British Medical Journal* 335, no. 7627 (November 2007): 951.

10. Brian Berman et al., Reviewing the Reviews, *International Journal of Technology Assessment in Health Care,* 17 (2001): 457–66.

11. For the facts about depression around the world, go to the World Health Organization's website on the matter: www.who.int/mediacentre/ factsheets/fs369/en/.

12. This section is adapted from my own blog posts at www.kellybroganmd. com. In particular, see "Have You Been Told It's All In Your Head? The New Biology of Mental Illness," September 25, 2014.

13. R. Mojtabai and M. Olfson, "Proportion of Antidepressants Prescribed without a Psychiatric Diagnosis Is Growing," *Health Affairs* (Millwood) 30, no. 8 (August 2011): 1434–42. doi: 10.1377/hlthaff.2010.1024. Also see: Nancy Shute, "Antidepressant Use Climbs, as Primary Care Doctors Do the Prescribing," National Public Radio, August 4, 2011, www.npr.org/ sections/health-shots/2011/08/06/138987152/antidepressant-use-climbs-as-primary-care-doctors-do-the-prescribing, accessed September 22, 2015.

14. See my blog post at www.kellybroganmd.com, "Antidepressants: No Diagnosis Needed," April 21, 2014.

15. Y. Takayanagi et al., "Antidepressant Use and Lifetime History of Mental Disorders in a Community Sample: Results from the Baltimore Epidemiologic Catchment Area Study," *Journal of Clinical Psychiatry* 76, no. 1 (January 2015): 40–44, doi: 10.4088/JCP.13m08824.

16. For a general review of the relationship between inflammation

and depression, see: A. H. Miller et al., "Inflammation and Its Discontents: The Role of Cytokines in the Pathophysiology of Major Depression," *Biol Psychiatry* 65, no. 9 (May 1, 2009): 732–41, doi: 10.1016/j.biopsych.2008.11.029. Also see: E. Haroon et al., "Psychoneuroimmunology Meets Neuropsychopharmacology: Translational Implications of the Impact of Inflammation on Behavior," *Neuropsychopharmacology* 37, no. 1 (January 2012): 137–62, doi: 10.1038/npp.2011.205.

17. R. Dantzer et al., "From Inflammation to Sickness and Depression: When the Immune System Subjugates the Brain," *Nat Rev Neurosci*, 9, no. 1 (January 2008): 46–56.

18. M. Udina et al., "Interferon-induced Depression in Chronic Hepatitis C: A Systematic Review and Meta-analysis," *J Clin Psychiatry* 73, no. 8 (August 2012): 1128–38, doi: 10.4088/JCP.12r07694. Also see: M. Alavi et al., "Effect of Pegylated Interferon-α-2a Treatment on Mental Health During Recent Hepatitis C Virus Infection," *J Gastroenterol Hepatol* 27, no. 5 (May 2012): 957–65, doi: 10.1111/j.1440-1746.2011.07035.x.

19. C. Andre et al., "Diet-induced Obesity Progressively Alters Cognition, Anxiety-like Behavior and Lipopolysaccharide-induced Depressive-like Behavior: Focus on Brain Indoleamine 2,3-dioxygenase Activation," *Brain Behav Immun* 41 (October 2014): 10–21, doi: 10.1016/j.bbi.2014.03.012.

20. A. Pan et al., "Bidirectional Association between Depression and Type 2 Diabetes Mellitus in Women," *Arch Intern Med* 170, no. 21 (November 22, 2010): 1884–91. doi: 10.1001/archinternmed.2010.356.

21. F. S. Luppino et al., "Overweight, Obesity, and Depression: A Systematic Review and Meta-analysis of Longitudinal Studies," *JAMA Psychiatry* 67, no. 3 (March 2010).

22. M. Berk et al., "So Depression Is an Inflammatory Disease, but Where Does the Inflammation Come From? *BMC Med* 11 (September 12, 2013): 200, doi: 10.1186/1741-7015-11-200.

23. G. Anderson et al., "Biological Phenotypes Underpin the Physio-somatic Symptoms of Somatization, Depression, and Chronic Fatigue Syndrome," *Acta Psychiatr Scand* 129, no. 2 (February 2014): 83–97, doi: 10.1111/acps.12182.

24. Ibid.

25. A. Louveau et al., "Structural and Functional Features of Central Nervous System Lymphatic Vessels," *Nature* 523, no. 7560 (July 16, 2015): 337–41, doi: 10.1038/nature14432.

26. For a general overview of the human microbiome, visit the home of the Human Microbiome Project at http://hmpdacc.org/overview/about.php.

27. To read about Hans Selye and the history or "birth of stress," go to the American Institute of Stress at www.stress.org.

28. Bruce S. McEwen and Eliot Stellar, "Stress and the Individual: Mechanisms Leading to Disease," *Arch Intern Med* 153, no. 18 (1993): 2093–2101, doi:10.1001/archinte.1993.00410180039004.

29. E. S. Wohleb et al., "Monocyte Trafficking to the Brain with Stress and Inflammation: a Novel Axis of Immune-to-brain Communication that Influences Mood and Behavior," *Front Neurosci* 8 (January 21, 2015): 447, doi: 10.3389/fnins.2014.00447.

30. R. L. O'Sullivan et al., "The Neuro-immuno-cutaneous-endocrine Network: Relationship of Mind and Skin," *Arch Dermatol* 134, no. 11 (November 1998): 1431–35.

31. Z. Durisko et al., "An Adaptationist Perspective on the Etiology of Depression," *J Affect Disord* 172C (September 28, 2014): 315–23, doi: 10.1016/j.jad.2014.09.032.

32. See my post at www.kellybroganmd.com, "A Model Consent Form for Psychiatric Drug Treatment," June 2, 2015.

33. J. Tiihonen et al., "Psychotropic Drugs and Homicide: a Prospective Cohort Study from Finland," *World Psychiatry* (2015), doi: 10.1002/wps.20220.

34. P. C. Gøtzsche et al., "Does Long Term Use of Psychiatric Drugs Cause More Harm than Good?" *BMJ* 350 (Mary 12, 2015): h2435, doi: 10.1136/bmj.h2435.

35. A. Amerio et al., "Are Antidepressants Mood Destabilizers?" *Psychiatry Res* 227, no. 2–3 (June 30, 2015): 374–75, doi: 10.1016/j.psychres.2015.03.028.

36. See my post at www.kellybroganmd.com, "Psych Meds Put 49 Million Americans at Risk for Cancer," May 5, 2015.

37. A. Amerio et al., "Carcinogenicity of Psychotropic Drugs: A Systematic Review of US Food and Drug Administration-required Preclinical in Vivo Studies," *Australian and New Zealand Journal of Psychiatry* 49, no. 8 (August 2015): 686–96, doi: 10.1177/0004867415582231.

38. N. Berry et al., "Catatonia and Other Psychiatric Symptoms with Vitamin B_{12} Deficiency," *Acta Psychiatr Scand* 108, no. 2 (August 2003): 156–59.

CHAPTER 2: TRUTH SERUM: COMING CLEAN ABOUT THE SEROTONIN MYTH

1. Julia Calderone, "The Rise of All-Purpose Antidepressants," *Scientific American* 24, no. 6 (October 16, 2014), www.scientificamerican.com/article/the-rise-of-all-purpose-antidepressants/.

2. Parts of this section are adapted from my post on Mercola.com, entitled "A Psychiatrist's Perspective on Using Drugs," January 16, 2014, http://articles.mercola.com/sites/articles/archive/2014/01/16/dr-brogan-on-depression.aspx, accessed September 21, 2015.

3. For a well-cited history on antidepressant use, see Robert Whitaker's *Anatomy of an Epidemic: Magic Bullets, Psychiatric Drugs, and the Astonishing Rise of Mental Illness in America* (New York: Crown, 2010). Also visit his website at www.MadinAmerica.com.

4. Ibid.

5. M. A. Posternak et al., "The Naturalistic Course of Unipolar Major Depression in the Absence of Somatic Therapy," *J Nerv Ment Dis* 194, no. 5 (May 2006): 324–29.

6. L. Cosgrove et al., "Financial Ties between DSM-IV Panel Members and the Pharmaceutical Industry," *Psychother Psychosom* 75, no. 3 (2006): 154–60.

7. To access a collection of Dr. Allen Frances's articles, see his posts at *Psychiatric Times*, www.psychiatrictimes.com/authors/allen-frances-md. Also check out his book, *Saving Normal: An Insider's Revolt Against Out-of-Control Psychiatric Diagnosis, DSM-5, Big Pharma, and the Medicalization of Ordinary Life* (New York: William Morrow, 2013). Also see: www.psychiatrictimes.com/authors/allen-frances-md#sthash.NJ03o7jI.dpuf.

8. Allen Frances, "The New Crisis of Confidence in Psychiatric Diagnosis," *Annals of Internal Medicine* 159, no. 3 (August 6, 2013): 221–22. Also see: Allen Frances's "The Past, Present and Future of Psychiatric Diagnosis," *World Psychiatry* 12, no. 2 (June 2013): 111–12.

9. Y. Takayanagi et al., "Antidepressant Use and Lifetime History of Mental Disorders in a Community Sample: Results from the Baltimore Epidemiologic Catchment Area Study," *Journal of Clinical Psychiatry* 76, no. 1 (January 2015): 40–44, doi: 10.4088/JCP.13m08824.

10. Peter Doshi, "No Correction, No Retraction, No Apology, No Comment: Paroxetine Trial Reanalysis Raises Questions about Institutional Responsibility," *BMJ* 351 (2015): h4629.

11. To access the actual lawsuit document, see www.justice.gov/sites/default/files/opa/legacy/2012/07/02/us-complaint.pdf.

12. J. Moncrieff and D. Cohen, "Do Antidepressants Cure or Create Abnormal Brain States? *PLoS Med* 3, no. 7 (July 2006): e240.

13. Parts of this section are adapted from my post on Mercola.com, entitled "A Psychiatrist's Perspective on Using Drugs," January 16, 2014, http://articles.mercola.com/sites/articles/archive/2014/01/16/dr-brogan-on-depression.aspx, accessed September 21, 2015.

14. See parts I and II of F. Lopez-Munoz et al., "Half a Century of Antidepressant Drugs: On the Clinical Introduction of Monoamine Oxidase Inhibitors, Tricyclics, and Tetracyclics. Monoamine Oxidase Inhibitors," *J Clin Psychopharmacol* 27, no. 6 (December 2007): 555–59. Also see: D. L. Davies and M. Shepherd, "Reserpine in the Treatment of Anxious and Depressed Patients," *Lancet* 269, no. 6881 (July 16, 1955): 117–20.

15. D. L. Davies and M. Shepherd, "Reserpine in the Treatment of Anxious and Depressed Patients," *Lancet* 269, no. 6881 (July 16, 1955): 117–20.

16. J. J. Schildkraut, "The Catecholamine Hypothesis of Affective Disorders: A review of Supporting Evidence. 1965," *J Neuropsychiatry Clin Neurosci* 7, no. 4 (Fall 1995): 524–33; discussion 523–24.

17. E. Castrén, "Is Mood Chemistry?" *Nat Rev Neurosci* 6, no. 3 (March 2005): 241–46.

18. R. H. Belmaker and G. Agam, "Major Depressive Disorder," *N Engl J Med* 358, no. 1 (January 2008): 55–68, doi: 10.1056/NEJMra073096.

19. K. S. Lam et al., "Neurochemical Correlates of Autistic Disorder: A Review of the Literature," *Res Dev Disabil* 27 (2006): 254–89. Also see: A. Abi-Dargham et al., "The Role of Serotonin in the Pathophysiology and Treatment of Schizophrenia," *J Neuropsychiatry Clin Neurosci* 9 (1997): 1–17.

20. Paul W. Andrews et al., "Is Serotonin an Upper or a Downer? The Evolution of the Serotonergic System and Its Role in Depression and the Antidepressant Response," *Neuroscience & Behavioral Reviews* 51 (April 2015): 164–88. To learn more about Paul Andrews's research and to retrieve a selected list of his publications, check out his website at www.science.mcmaster.ca/pnb/andrews.

21. McMaster University. "Science behind commonly used anti-depressants appears to be backwards, researchers say." ScienceDaily. www.sciencedaily.com/releases/2015/02/150217114119.htm, accessed September 22, 2015.

22. E. Castrén, "Is Mood Chemistry?" *Nat Rev Neurosci* 6, no. 3 (March, 2005): 241–46.

23. R. H. Belmaker and G. Agam, "Major Depressive Disorder," *N Engl J Med* 358, no. 1 (January 2008): 55–68, doi: 10.1056/NEJMra073096.

24. Daniel Carlat, *Unhinged: The Trouble with Psychiatry—A Doctor's Revelations about a Profession in Crisis* (New York: Free Press, 2010).

25. Peter Breggin and David Cohen, *Your Drug May Be Your Problem: How and Why to Stop Taking Psychiatric Medications* (New York: Da Capo Press, 1999).

26. Avshalom Caspi et al., "Influence of Life Stress on Depression: Moderation by a Polymorphism in the 5-HTT Gene," *Science* (July 18, 2003): 386–89.

27. N. Risch et al., "Interaction between the Serotonin Transporter Gene (5-HTTLPR), Stressful Life Events, and Risk of Depression: A Meta-analysis," *JAMA* 301, no. 23 (June 17, 2009): 2462–71, doi: 10.1001/jama.2009.878.

28. See my post at www.kellybroganmd.com, "Depression: It's Not Your Serotonin," January 4, 2015, http://kellybroganmd.com/article/depression-serotonin/.

29. To read more about Daniel Carlat's work and publications, go to www.danielcarlat.com.

30. Jeffrey R. Lacasse and Jonathan Leo, "Serotonin and Depression: A Disconnect between the Advertisements and the Scientific Literature," *PLoS Med* 2, no. 12 (November 8, 2005): e392, doi:10.1371/journal.pmed.0020392. Also see their latest update to this paper in "Antidepressants and the Chemical Imbalance Theory of Depression: A Reflection and Update on the Discourse," *Behavior Therapist* 38, no. 7 (October 2015): 206. This is a publication by the Association for Behavioral and Cognitive Therapies.

31. E. Murray et al., "Direct-to-consumer Advertising: Physicians' Views of Its Effects on Quality of Care and the Doctor-patient Relationship," *J Am Board Fam Pract* 16, no. 6 (November–December, 2003): 513–24.

32. R. J. Avery et al., "The Impact of Direct-to-consumer Television and Magazine Advertising on Antidepressant Use," *J Health Econ* 31, no. 5 (September 2012): 705–18, doi: 10.1016/j.jhealeco.2012.05.002.

33. Tracy Staton, "Pharma's Ad Spend Vaults to $4.5B, with Big Spender Pfizer Leading the Way," March 25, 2015, www.fiercepharmamarketing.com/story/pharmas-ad-spend-vaults-45b-big-spender-pfizer-leading-way/2015-03-25.

34. Jeffrey R. Lacasse and Jonathan Leo, "Serotonin and Depression: A Disconnect between the Advertisements and the Scientific Literature," *PLoS Med* 2, no. 12 (November 8, 2005): e392, doi:10.1371/journal.pmed.0020392.

35. E. S. Valenstein, *Blaming the Brain: The Truth about Drugs and Mental Health* (New York: Free Press, 1998), p. 292.

36. Brendan L. Smith, "Inappropriate Prescribing," *Monitor on Psychology*, a publication by the American Psychological Association, vol. 43, no. 6 (June 2012): 36, www.apa.org/monitor/2012/06/prescribing.aspx. Also see: Carolyn C. Ross's post "Do Antidepressants Really Work?" *Psychology Today*, February 20, 2012, www.psychologytoday.com/blog/real-healing/201202/do-anti-depressants-really-work.

37. "The Other Drug War: Big Pharma's 625 Washington Lobbysits," by

Citizen.org, July 23, 2001, www.citizen.org/documents/pharmadrugwar. PDF. For an overview of the corruption within Big Pharma as it relates with data, see Ben Wolford's cover story for *Newsweek* magazine, "Big Pharma Plays Hide-the-Ball With Data," November 13, 2014.

38. Ibid.

39. E. H. Turner et al., "Selective Publication of Antidepressant Trials and Its Influence on Apparent Efficacy," *N Engl J Med* 358, no. 3 (January 17, 2008): 252–60, doi: 10.1056/NEJMsa065779.

40. M. Fava et al., "A Comparison of Mirtazapine and Nortriptyline Following Two Consecutive Failed Medication Treatments for Depressed Outpatients: A STAR*D Report," *Am J Psychiatry* 163, no. 7 (July 2006): 1161–72.

41. John T. Aquino, "Whistleblower Claims Forest Bribed Study's Investigator to Favor Celexa," Bloomberg Bureau of National Affairs, February 1, 2012, www.bna.com/whistleblower-claims-forest-n12884907568/.

42. See www.fda.gov/ICECI/CriminalInvestigations/ucm245543.htm.

43. Irving Kirsch and Guy Sapirstein, "Listening to Prozac but Hearing Placebo: A Meta-analysis of Antidepressant Medication," *Prevention & Treatment* 1, no. 2 (June 1998).

44. Irving Kirsch et al., "Initial Severity and Antidepressant Benefits: A Meta-Analysis of Data Submitted to the Food and Drug Administration," *PLoS Med* 5, no. 2 (2008): e45, doi: 10.1371/journal.pmed.0050045.

45. Irving Kirsch, "Challenging Received Wisdom: Antidepressants and the Placebo Effect," *Mcgill J Med* 11, no. 2 (November 2008): 219–22.

46. To learn more about Dr. Kirsch's work and publications, go to his site at the Program in Placebo Studies & Therapeutic Encounter (PiPS), which is part of Harvard Medical School, http://programinplacebostudies.org/about/people/irving-kirsch/.

47. B. R. Rutherford et al., "The Role of Patient Expectancy in Placebo and Nocebo Effects in Antidepressant Trials," *J Clin Psychiatry* 75, no. 10 (October 2014): 1040–46, doi: 10.4088/JCP.13m08797.

48. To learn more about the work of Dr. David Healy, go to his site at http://davidhealy.org/.

49. See www.MadinAmerica.com.

50. For a list of studies supporting the facts of antidepressant use both in the short and long term, see Whitaker's "Antidepressants/Depression" page on his site: www.madinamerica.com/mia-manual/antidepressantsdepression/.

51. C. Ronalds et al., "Outcome of Anxiety and Depressive Disorders in Primary Care," *Br J Psychiatry* 171 (November 1997): 427–33.

52. D. Goldberg et al., "The Effects of Detection and Treatment on the Outcome of Major Depression in Primary Care: A Naturalistic Study in 15 Cities," *Br J Gen Pract* 48, no. 437 (December 1998): 1840–44.

53. Thomas J. Moore et al., "Prescription Drugs Associated with Reports of Violence Towards Others," *PLoS One* 5, no. 12 (December 15 2010): e15337.

54. See: www.madinamerica.com/mia-manual/antidepressantsdepression/.

55. See: www.ncbi.nlm.nih.gov/books/NBK54348/.

56. A. Louveau et al., "Structural and Functional Features of Central Nervous System Lymphatic Vessels," *Nature* 523, no. 7560 (July 16, 2015): 337-41, doi: 10.1038/nature14432.

57. Alexander Schaefer, et al., "Serotonergic Modulation of Intrinsic Functional Connectivity," *Current Biology* 24, no. 19 (September 2014): 2314-8, doi: 10.1016/j.cub.2014.08.024.

58. S. E. Hyman and E. J. Nestler, "Initiation and Adaptation: A Paradigm for Understanding Psychotropic Drug Action," *Am J Psychiatry* 153, no. 2 (February 1996): 151–62.

59. P. W. Andrews et al., "Blue Again: Perturbational Effects of Antidepressants Suggest Monoaminergic Homeostasis in Major Depression," *Front Psychol* 2 (July 7, 2011): 159, doi: 10.3389/fpsyg.2011.00159.

60. Ibid.

61. E. M. van Weel-Baumgarten et al., "Treatment of Depression Related to Recurrence: 10-Year Follow-up in General Practice," *J Clin Pharm Ther* 25, no. 1 (February 2000): 61–66.

62. A. C. Viguera et al., "Discontinuing Antidepressant Treatment in Major Depression," *Harv Rev Psychiatry* 5, no. 6 (March-April 1998): 293–306.

63. See: www.madinamerica.com/wp-content/uploads/2011/11/Can-long-term-andtidepressant-use-be-depressogenic.pdf.

64. Phil Hickey, "Antidepressants Make Things Worse in the Long Term," Behaviorism and Mental Health blog post on April 8, 2014, www.behaviorismandmentalhealth.com/2014/04/08/antidepressants-make-things-worse-in-the-long-term/.

65. Robert Whitaker, *Anatomy of an Epidemic: Magic Bullets, Psychiatric Drugs, and the Astonishing Rise of Mental Illness in America* (New York: Crown, 2010), pp. 169–70.

66. See: www.madinamerica.com/2015/02/stopping-ssri-antidepressants-can-cause-long-intense-withdrawal-problems/.

67. G. Chouinard and V. A. Chouinard, "New Classification of Selective Serotonin Reuptake Inhibitor Withdrawal," *Psychother Psychosom* 84, no. 2 (February 21, 2015): 63–71.

68. This language comes from my post on MadinAmerica.com, "Depression: It's Not Your Serotonin," December 30, 2014, www.madinamerica. com/2014/12/depression-serotonin/.

69. M. Babyak et al., Exercise Treatment for Major Depression: Maintenance of Therapeutic Benefit at 10 Months," *Psychosom Med* 62, no. 5 (September–October 2000): 633–38.

CHAPTER 3: THE NEW BIOLOGY OF DEPRESSION

1. O. Köhler et al., "Effect of Anti-inflammatory Treatment on Depression, Depressive Symptoms, and Adverse Effects: A Systematic Review and Meta-analysis of Randomized Clinical Trials," *JAMA Psychiatry* 71, no. 12 (December 1, 2014): 1381–91, doi: 10.1001/jamapsychiatry.2014.1611.

2. E. Haroon et al., "Psychoneuroimmunology Meets Neuropsychopharmacology: Translational Implications of the Impact of Inflammation on Behavior," *Neuropsychopharmacology* 37, no. 1 (January 2012): 137–62, doi: 10.1038/npp.2011.205.

3. Norbert Müller, "Immunology of Major Depression," *Neuroimmunomodulation* 21, no. 2–3 (2014): 123–30. doi: 10.1159/000356540.

4. S. M. Gibney and H. A. Drexhage, "Evidence for a Dysregulated Immune System in the Etiology of Psychiatric Disorders," *J Neuroimmune Pharmacol* 8, no. 4 (September 2013): 900–920, doi: 10.1007/s11481-013-9462-8.

5. A. C. Logan et al., "Natural Environments, Ancestral Diets, and Microbial Ecology: Is There a Modern "Paleo-deficit Disorder? Part I" *J Physiol Anthropol* 35, no. 1 (2015): 1. Published online January 31, 2015, doi: 10.1186/s40101-015-0041-y.

6. Paula A. Garay and A. Kimberley McAllister, "Novel Roles for Immune Molecules in Neural Development: Implications for Neurodevelopmental Disorders," *Front Synaptic Neurosci* 2 (2010): 136, doi: 10.3389/fnsyn.2010.00136.

7. A. Louveau et al., "Structural and Functional Features of Central Nervous System Lymphatic Vessels," *Nature* 523, no. 7560 (July 16, 2015): 337–41, doi: 10.1038/nature14432.

8. C. Martin et al., "The Inflammatory Cytokines: Molecular Biomarkers for Major Depressive Disorder?" *Biomark Med* 9, no. 2 (2015): 169–80, doi: 10.2217/bmm.14.29.

9. J. Dahl et al., "The Plasma Levels of Various Cytokines Are Increased During Ongoing Depression and Are Reduced to Normal Levels After Recovery," *Psychoneuroendocrinology* 45 (July 2014): 77–86, doi: 10.1016/j. psyneuen.2014.03.019. Also see: S. Alesci et al., "Major Depression Is

Associated with Significant Diurnal Elevations in Plasma Interleukin-6 Levels, a Shift of Its Circadian Rhythm, and Loss of Physiological Complexity in Its Secretion: Clinical Implications," *J Clin Endocrinol Metab* 90, no. 5 (May 2005): 2522–30.

10. J. A. Pasco et al., "Association of High-sensitivity C-reactive Protein with de novo Major Depression," *Br J Psychiatry* 197, no. 5 (November 2010): 372-7, doi: 10.1192/bjp.bp.109.076430.

11. C. Hoyo-Becerra et al., "Insights from Interferon-α-related Depression for the Pathogenesis of Depression Associated with Inflammation," *Brain Behav Immun* 42 (November 2014): 222–31, doi: 10.1016/j.bbi.2014.06.200.

12. S. C. Segerstrom and G. E. Miller, "Psychological Stress and the Human Immune System: a Meta-analytic Study of 30 Years of Inquiry," *Psychol Bull* 130, no. 4 (July 2004): 601–30.

13. L. A. Carvalho et al., "Inflammatory Activation Is Associated with a Reduced Glucocorticoid Receptor alpha/beta Expression Ratio in Monocytes of Inpatients with Melancholic Major Depressive Disorder," *Transl Psychiatry* 4 (January 14, 2014): e344, doi: 10.1038/tp.2013.118.

14. O. Köhler et al., "Effect of Anti-inflammatory Treatment on Depression, Depressive Symptoms, and Adverse Effects: A Systematic Review and Meta-analysis of Randomized Clinical Trials," *JAMA Psychiatry* 71, no. 12 (December 1, 2014): 1381–91, doi: 10.1001/jamapsychiatry.2014.1611.

15. J. J. Yu et al., "Chronic Supplementation of Curcumin Enhances the Efficacy of Antidepressants in Major Depressive Disorder: A Randomized, Double-Blind, Placebo-Controlled Pilot Study," *J Clin Psychopharmacol* 35, no. 4 (August 2015): 406–10, doi: 10.1097/JCP.0000000000000352.

16. M. Maes et al., "The Gut-brain Barrier in Major Depression: Intestinal Mucosal Dysfunction with an Increased Translocation of LPS from Gram Negative Enterobacteria (Leaky Gut) Plays a Role in the Inflammatory Pathophysiology of Depression," *Neuro Endocrinol Lett* 29, no. 1 (February 2008): 117–24.

17. M. Berk et al., "So Depression Is an Inflammatory Disease, but Where Does the Inflammation Come From?," *BMC Med* 11 (September 12, 2013): 200, doi: 10.1186/1741-7015-11-200.

18. Y. Gao et al., "Depression as a Risk Factor for Dementia and Mild Cognitive Impairment: a Meta-analysis of Longitudinal Studies," *Int J Geriatr Psychiatry* 28, no. 5 (May 2013): 441–49, doi: 10.1002/gps.3845. Epub July 19, 2012. Also see: A. C. Bested et al., "Intestinal Microbiota, Probiotics and Mental Health: from Metchnikoff to Modern Advances: Part II—Contemporary Contextual Research," *Gut Pathog* 5, no. 1 (March 14, 2013): 3, doi: 10.1186/1757-4749-5-3.

19. T. C. Theoharis, "On the Gut Microbiome-Brain Axis and Altruism," Editorial for *Clinical Therapeutics*, 37, no. 5 (2015).

20. T. G. Dinan and J. F. Cryan, "Regulation of the Stress Response by the Gut Microbiota: Implications for Psychoneuroendocrinology," *Psychoneuroendocrinology* 37, no. 9 (September 2012): 1369–78, doi: 10.1016/j.psyneuen.2012.03.007.

21. For a great overview about the human microbiome, see Peter Andrey Smith's "Can the Bacteria in Your Gut Explain Your Mood?" *New York Times* magazine, June 23, 2105, www.nytimes.com/2015/06/28/magazine/can-the-bacteria-in-your-gut-explain-your-mood.html?smid=fb-nytimes&smtyp=cur&_r=1.

22. P. Bercik et al., "Chronic Gastrointestinal Inflammation Induces Anxiety-like Behavior and Alters Central Nervous System Biochemistry in Mice," *Gastroenterology* 139, no. 6 (December 2010): 2102–112.e1, doi: 10.1053/j.gastro.2010.06.063.

23. P. Bercik et al., "The Intestinal Microbiota Affect Central Levels of Brain-derived Neurotropic Factor and Behavior in Mice," *Gastroenterology* 141, no. 2 (August 14 2011): 599–609, 609.e1-3, doi: 10.1053/j.gastro.2011.04.052.

24. M. J. Friedrich, "Unraveling the Influence of Gut Microbes on the Mind," *JAMA* 313, no. 17 (2015): 1699–1701, doi:10.1001/jama.2015.2159.

25. Ibid.

26. Daniel Erny et al., "Host Microbiota Constantly Control Maturation and Function of Microglia in the CNS," *Nature Neuroscience* 18 (2015): 965–77, doi:10.1038/nn.4030. Also see: Y. E. Borre et al., "Microbiota and Neurodevelopmental Windows: Implications for Brain Disorders," *Trends Mol Med* 20, no. 9 (September 2014): 509–18. doi: 10.1016/j.molmed.2014.05.002.

27. M. B. Azad et al., "Gut Microbiota of Healthy Canadian Infants: Profiles by Mode of Delivery and Infant Diet at 4 Months," *CMAJ* 185, no. 5 (March 19, 2013): 385–94, doi: 10.1503/cmaj.121189.

28. *Canadian Medical Association Journal.* "Infant gut microbiota influenced by cesarean section and breastfeeding practices; may impact long-term health." ScienceDaily. www.sciencedaily.com/releases/2013/02/130211134842.htm, accessed September 23, 2015.

29. Martin J. Blaser, *Missing Microbes: How the Overuse of Antibiotics Is Fueling Our Modern Plagues* (New York: Henry Holt and Co., 2014).

30. M. G. Dominguez-Bello, et al., "Delivery Mode Shapes the Acquisition and Structure of the Initial Microbiota Across Multiple Body Habitats in Newborns," *Proc Natl Acad Sci USA* 107, no. 26 (June 29, 2010): 11971–75.

31. A. C. Logan et al., "Natural Environments, Ancestral Diets, and Microbial Ecology: Is There a Modern "Paleo-deficit Disorder? Part I," *J Physiol Anthropol* 35, no. 1 (2015): 1. Published online January 31, 2015, doi: 10.1186/s40101-015-0041-y. Also see Part II: www.ncbi.nlm.nih.gov/pmc/articles/PMC4353476/.

32. S. L. Schnorr et al., "Gut Microbiome of the Hadza Hunter-gatherers," *Nat Commun* 5 (April 15, 2014): 3654, doi: 10.1038/ncomms4654. Also see: "Some Indigenous People from the Amazon Have the Richest and Most Diverse Microbiota Ever Recorded in Humans," article posted May 20, 2015, by Gut Microbiota Watch Organization at www.gutmicrobiotawatch.org.

33. For more about Dr. William Parker's work and a list of publications, go to http://surgery.duke.edu/faculty/details/0115196.

34. A. C. Logan et al., "Natural Environments, Ancestral Diets, and Microbial Ecology: Is There a Modern "Paleo-deficit Disorder? Part I," *J Physiol Anthropol* 35, no. 1 (2015): 1. Published online January 31, 2015 doi: 10.1186/s40101-015-0041-y.

35. Ibid.

36. Peter J. Turnbaugh et al., "A Core Gut Microbiome in Obese and Lean Twins," *Nature* 457 (January 22, 2009): 480–84, doi:10.1038/nature07540. Also see: Peter J. Turnbaugh et al., "The Effect of Diet on the Human Gut Microbiome: A Metagenomic Analysis in Humanized Gnotobiotic Mice," *Sci Transl Med* 1, no. 6 (November 11, 2009): 6ra14, doi: 10.1126/scitranslmed.3000322.

37. A. C. Bested et al., "Intestinal Microbiota, Probiotics and Mental Health: from Metchnikoff to Modern Advances: Part II—Contemporary Contextual Research," *Gut Pathog* 5, no. 1 (March 14, 2013): 3, doi: 10.1186/1757-4749-5-3.

38. M. Hadjivassiliou et al., "Gluten Sensitivity as a Neurological Illness," *J Neurol Neurosurg Psychiatry* 72, no. 5 (May 2002): 560–63.

39. For a comprehensive discussion about the role of gluten in brain pathology, as well as a synthesis of the latest research, see Dr. David Perlmutter's *Grain Brain: The Surprising Truth about Wheat, Carbs, and Sugar . . . Your Brain's Silent Killers* (New York: Little, Brown, 2013). Also see: D. B. Shor et al., "Gluten Sensitivity in Multiple Sclerosis: Experimental Myth or Clinical Truth?" *Ann N Y Acad Sci* 1173 (September 2009): 343–49.

40. D. Bernardo et al., "Is Gliadin Really Safe for Non-coeliac Individuals? Production of Interleukin 15 in Biopsy Culture from Non-coeliac Individuals Challenged with Gliadin Peptides," *Gut* 56, no. 6 (June 2007): 889–90.

41. For a great review and collection of references about the effects of glyphosate, see Dr. Joseph Mercola's "Research Reveals Previously Unknown Pathway by which Glyphosate Wrecks Health," posting on Mercola.com on May 14, 2013, http://articles.mercola.com/sites/articles/archive/2013/05/14/glyphosate.aspx.

42. J. Suez et al., "Artificial Sweeteners Induce Glucose Intolerance by Altering the Gut Microbiota," *Nature* 514, no. 7521 (October 9, 2014): 181–86, doi: 10.1038/nature13793.

CHAPTER 4: THE GREAT PSYCHIATRIC PRETENDERS

1. P. Caturegli et al., "Hashimoto's Thyroiditis: Celebrating the Centennial through the Lens of the Johns Hopkins Hospital Surgical Pathology Records," *Thyroid* 23, no. 2 (February 2013): 142–50, doi: 10.1089/thy.2012.0554.

2. For a comprehensive list of Dr. Gold's publications, go to www.drmarkgold.com/dr-mark-s-gold-addiction-medicine-books-and-publications/.

3. D. Degner et al., "Association between Autoimmune Thyroiditis and Depressive Disorder in Psychiatric Outpatients," *Eur Arch Psychiatry Clin Neurosci* 265, no. 1 (February 2015): 67–72, doi: 10.1007/s00406-014-0529-1.

4. For a summary of the research on thyroid and symptoms of depression, go to www.kellybroganmd.com and read the following posts: "Thyroid: What's Mental Health Got to Do with It" (July 14, 2014); "New Habits Die Hard—Dessicated Thyroid Treatment" (December 11, 2013); and "Is Thyroid Hormone Dangerous for Psych Patients?" (March 24, 2015).

5. Troy Brown, "The 10 Most-Prescribed and Top-Selling Medications," WebMD post, May 8, 2015, www.webmd.com/news/20150508/most-prescribed-top-selling-drugs.

6. C. Sategna-Guidetti et al., "Prevalence of Thyroid Disorders in Untreated Adult Celiac Disease Patients and Effect of Gluten Withdrawal: An Italian Multicenter Study," *Am J Gastroenterol* 96, no. 3 (March 2001): 751–57.

7. For a synthesis of the research showing the relationship between fluoride and thyroid dysfunction, go to http://fluoridealert.org/issues/health/thyroid/.

8. See my post at www.kellybroganmd.com, "Pheromones Missing From That Similac?" November 13, 2014, http://kellybroganmd.com/snippet/pheromones-missing-similac/.

9. Ibid.

10. For a general overview of the relationship between blood sugar issues, diabetes, and depression, see www.nimh.nih.gov/health/publications/depression-and-diabetes/index.shtml.

11. W. K. Kim et al., "Depression and Its Comorbid Conditions More Serious in Women than in Men in the United States," *J Women's Health* (Larchmt) (July 1, 2015).

CHAPTER 5: WHY BODY LOTIONS, TAP WATER, AND OTC PAIN RELIEVERS SHOULD COME WITH NEW WARNING LABELS

1. For a synthesis of the research on the relationship between the Pill and psychiatric disorders, see my post at www.kellybroganmd.com, "Is the Pill Changing Your Brain?" April 28, 2015, http://kellybroganmd. com/snippet/oral-contraceptives/. Also see: "That Naughty Little Pill," post on MadinAmerica.com, February 8, 2013, www.madinamerica. com/2013/02/that-naughty-little-pill/.

2. Some of the language in this section reflects that of my post "That Naughty Little Pill," on MadinAmerica.com, February 8, 2013, http:// www.madinamerica.com/2013/02/that-naughty-little-pill/.

3. K. A. Oinonen and D. J. Mazmanian, "To What Extent Do Oral Contraceptives Influence Mood and Affect?," *J Affect Disord* 70, no. 3 (August 2002): 229–40.

4. KellyBroganMD.com, "That Naughty Little Pill," post on MadinAmerica. com, February 8, 2013, www.madinamerica.com/2013/02/ that-naughty-little-pill/.

5. T. Piltonen et al., "Oral, Transdermal and Vaginal Combined Contraceptives Induce an Increase in Markers of Chronic Inflammation and Impair Insulin Sensitivity in Young Healthy Normal-weight Women: A Randomized Study," *Hum Reprod* 27, no. 10 (October 2012): 3046–56, doi: 10.1093/humrep/des225.

6. C. Panzer et al., "Impact of Oral Contraceptives on Sex Hormone-binding Globulin and Androgen Levels: A Retrospective Study in Women with Sexual Dysfunction," *J Sex Med* 3, no. 1 (January 2006): 104–13.

7. F. Zal et al., "Effect of Vitamin E and C Supplements on Lipid Peroxidation and GSH Dependent Antioxidant Enzyme Status in the Blood of Women Consuming Oral Contraceptives," *Contraception* 86, no. 1 (July 2012): 62-66, doi: 10.1016/j.contraception.2011.11.006.

8. P. R. Palan et al., "Effects of Oral, Vaginal, and Transdermal Hormonal Contraception On Serum Levels of Coenzyme Q(10), Vitamin E, and Total Antioxidant Activity," *Obstet Gynecol Int* (2010): pii: 925635, doi: 10.1155/2010/925635.

9. O. Akinloye et al., "Effects of Contraceptives on Serum Trace Elements, Calcium and Phosphorus Levels," *West Indian Med J* 60, no. 3 (June 2011): 308–15. For more details about the Pill's effects, especially as it relates to

the brain, see my post at www.kellybroganmd.com, "Is the Pill Changing Your Brain?" April 28, 2015.

10. This section is adapted from a post written by Sayer Ji and me at www. GreenMedInfo.com, "Cracking the Cholesterol Myth: How Statins Harm the Body and Mind," February 27, 2015, www.greenmedinfo.com/blog/ cracking-cholesterol-myth-how-statins-harm-body-and-mind?page=1#!.

11. "ACC/AHA Publish New Guideline for Management of Blood Cholesterol," American Heart Association, November 12, 2013, http://newsroom.heart.org/news/ acc-aha-publish-new-guideline-for-management-of-blood-cholesterol.

12. David M. Diamond and Uffe Ravnskov, "How Statistical Deception Created the Appearance that Statins Are Safe and Effective in Primary and Secondary Prevention of Cardiovascular Disease," *Expert Review of Clinical Pharmacology* 8, no. 2 (2015): 201, doi: 10.1586/17512433.2015.1012494.

13. For a brief general overview about the relationship between low cholesterol and depression, see Dr. James M. Greenblatt's post on *Psychology Today*, "Low Cholesterol and Its Psychological Effects," June 10, 2011, www.psychologytoday. com/blog/the-breakthrough-depression-solution/201106/ low-cholesterol-and-its-psychological-effects.

14. The next several paragraphs are adapted from my post "Luscious Lipids" on MadinAmerica.com, January 20, 2013, www.madinamerica. com/2013/01/luscious-lipids/.

15. For an overview of dietary fat's story in our lives and Ancel Keys's influence, see the cover story of *Time* magazine by Brian Shilhavy, "Ending the War on Fat," June 12, 2014.

16. I. Björkhem and S. Meaney, "Brain Cholesterol: Long Secret Life Behind a Barrier," *Arterioscler Thromb Vasc Biol* 24, no. 5 (May 2004): 806–15.

17. H. Kunugi et al., "Low Serum Cholesterol in Suicide Attempters," *Biol Psychiatry* 41, no. 2 (January 15, 1997): 196–200.

18. C. J. Glueck et al., "Hypocholesterolemia and Affective Disorders," *Am J Med Sci* 308, no. 4 (October 1994): 218–25.

19. E. C. Suarez, "Relations of Trait Depression and Anxiety to Low Lipid and Lipoprotein Concentrations in Healthy Young Adult Women," *Psychosom Med* 61, no. 3 (May-June 1999): 273–79.

20. V. W. Henderson et al., "Serum Lipids and Memory in a Population Based Cohort of Middle Age Women," *J Neurol Neurosurg Psychiatry* 74, no. 11 (November 2003): 1530–35.

21. H. Zhang et al., "Discontinuation of Statins in Routine Care Settings: A

Cohort Study," *Ann Intern Med* 158, no. 7 (April 2, 2013): 526–34, doi: 10.7326/0003-4819-158-7-201304020-00004.

22. A. L. Culver et al., "Statin Use and Risk of Diabetes Mellitus in Postmenopausal Women in the Women's Health Initiative," *Arch Intern Med* 172, no. 2 (January 23, 2012): 144–52, doi: 10.1001/archinternmed.2011.625.

23. This section is adapted from my post "Vitamin B$_{12}$ and Brain Health" at www.kellybroganmd.com, February 7, 2014, http://kellybroganmd.com/article/b12-deficiency-brain-health/.

24. N. Berry et al., "Catatonia and Other Psychiatric Symptoms with Vitamin B$_{12}$ Deficiency," *Acta Psychiatr Scand* 108, no. 2 (August 2003): 156–59.

25. J. R. Lam et al., "Proton Pump Inhibitor and Histamine 2 Receptor Antagonist Use and Vitamin B$_{12}$ Deficiency," *JAMA* 310, no. 22 (December 11, 2013): 2435–42, doi: 10.1001/jama.2013.280490.

26. For a good overview about the history and dangers of Tylenol, see Dr. Micozzi's post at Insiders' Cures, "Mainstream Press Finally Catches Wind of Tylenol's Dangers," March 30, 2015, http://drmicozzi.com/mainstream-press-finally-catches-wind-of-tylenols-dangers. Also see my post at kellybrogan.com, "Tylenol Numbing You Out?" April 30, 2015.

27. G. R. Durso, et al., "Over-the-Counter Relief From Pains and Pleasures Alike: Acetaminophen Blunts Evaluation Sensitivity to Both Negative and Positive Stimuli," *Psychol Sci* 26, no. 6 (June 2015): 750–58, doi: 10.1177/0956797615570366.

28. T. Christian Miller and Jeff Gerth, "Behind the Numbers," ProPublica, September 20, 2013, www.propublica.org/article/tylenol-mcneil-fda-behind-the-numbers.

29. R. E. Brandlistuen et al., "Prenatal Paracetamol Exposure and Child Neurodevelopment: A Sibling-controlled Cohort Study," *Int J Epidemiol* 42, no. 6 (December 2013): 1702–13, doi: 10.1093/ije/dyt183.

30. Z. Liew et al., "Acetaminophen Use During Pregnancy, Behavioral Problems, and Hyperkinetic Disorders," *JAMA Pediatr* 168, no. 4 (April 2014): 313–20, doi: 10.1001/jamapediatrics.2013.4914.

31. E. Roberts et al., "Paracetamol: Not as Safe as We Thought? A Systematic Literature Review of Observational Studies," *Ann Rheum Dis* (March 2, 2015), pii: annrheumdis-2014-206914, doi: 10.1136/annrheumdis-2014-206914.

32. European League Against Rheumatism. "Non-steroidal anti-inflammatory drugs inhibit ovulation after just 10 days." ScienceDaily, June 11, 2015. www.sciencedaily.com/releases/2015/06/150611082124.htm, accessed September 23, 2015.

33. D. Y. Graham et al., "Visible Small-intestinal Mucosal Injury in Chronic NSAID Users," *Clin Gastroenterol Hepatol* 3, no. 1 (January 2005): 55–59.

34. G. Sigthorsson et al., "Intestinal Permeability and Inflammation in Patients on NSAIDs," *Gut* 43, no. 4 (October 1998): 506–11.

35. See my post on Mercola.com, "Psychoneuroimmunology—How Inflammation Affects Your Mental Health," April 17, 2014, http://articles. mercola.com/sites/articles/archive/2014/04/17/psychoneuroimmunology-inflammation.aspx#_edn29.

36. European League Against Rheumatism. "Non-steroidal anti-inflammatory drugs inhibit ovulation after just 10 days." ScienceDaily, June 11, 2015. www.sciencedaily.com/releases/2015/06/150611082124.htm, accessed September 23, 2015.

37. G. Ozgoli, M. Goli, and F. Moattar, "Comparison of Effects of Ginger, Mefenamic Acid, and Ibuprofen on Pain in Women with Primary Dysmenorrhea," *J Altern Complement Med* 15, no. 2 (February 13, 2009): 129-32. See more at: http://www.greenmedinfo.com/blog/ibuprofen-kills-more-pain-so-what-alternatives?page=2#_ftn7. Also see: Vilai Kuptniratsaikul et al., "Efficacy and Safety of Curcuma Domestica Extracts in Patients with Knee Osteoarthritis," *Int J Mol Med* 25, no. 5 (May 2010): 729-34. See more at: http://www.greenmedinfo.com/blog/turmeric-extract-puts-drugs-knee-osteoarthritis-shame?page=2#sthash.gQAULVLl.dpuf.

38. A. L. Choi et al., "Developmental Fluoride Neurotoxicity: A Systematic Review and Meta-analysis," *Environ Health Perspect* 120, no. 10 (October 2012): 1362–68, doi: 10.1289/ehp.1104912.

39. See Jeremy Seifert's *Our Daily Dose*, a film about fluoridation. You can view it on YouTube at https://youtu.be/bZ6enuCZOA8. Also see my post "Are You Fluoridated," October 26, 2015, http://kellybroganmd.com/snippet/are-you-fluoridated/.

40. To access studies and facts about fluoride, go to the Fluoride Action Network website, http://fluoridealert.org/issues/health/brain/.

41. J. Luke, "Fluoride Deposition in the Aged Human Pineal Gland," *Caries Res* 35, no. 2 (March-April 2001): 125–28.

42. Check out Dr. Michael Ruscio's article and video on this matter, "Does Fluoride Cause Hypothyroidism?," at http://drruscio.com/fluoride-cause-hypothyroid/.

43. S. Peckham, D. Lowery, and S. Spencer, "Are Fluoride Levels in Drinking Water Associated with Hypothyroidism Prevalence in England? A Large Observational Study of GP Practice Data and Fluoride Levels in Drinking Water," *J Epidemiol Community Health* 69, no. 7 (July 2015): 619-24. doi: 10.1136/jech-2014-204971.

44. See my post at www.kellybrogan.com, "Will You Wait? Protect Yourself Now," November 4, 2014, http://kellybroganmd.com/snippet/will-wait-protect-now/.

45. R. U. Halden, "Epistemology of Contaminants of Emerging Concern and Literature Meta-analysis," *J Hazard Mater* 282 (January 2015): 2–9, doi: 10.1016/j.jhazmat.2014.08.074.

46. I. A. Lang et al., "Association of Urinary Bisphenol A Concentration with Medical Disorders and Laboratory Abnormalities in Adults," *JAMA* 300, no. 11 (September 2008): 1303–10, doi: 10.1001/jama.300.11.1303.

47. Jenna Bilbrey, "BPA-Free Plastic Containers May Be Just as Hazardous," *Scientific American*, August 11, 2014, www.scientificamerican.com/article/bpa-free-plastic-containers-may-be-just-as-hazardous/.

48. To access a user-friendly comprehensive resource center on the effects of vaccines and, in particular, the reporting of adverse reactions, visit the National Vaccine Information Center at http://medalerts.org/. I have written extensively on my concerns about vaccines, especially in vulnerable populations. I invite you to visit my website and use its search functionality to read more about my stand on vaccines and the supporting studies.

49. See my post "A Scientist Speaks: Senate Bill 277 in California" at www.kellybroganmd.com, May 7, 2015, http://kellybroganmd.com/article/scientist-speaks-senate-bill-277-california/.

50. To access the work of Dr. Gregory Poland and the Vaccine Research Group of the Mayo Clinic, go to www.mayo.edu/research/labs/vaccines/overview.

51. Donald L. Barlett and James B. Steele, "Deadly Medicine," *Vanity Fair,* January 2011.

52. To get the details on this story, see "Obama Grants Immunity to CDC Whistleblower on Measles Vaccine Link to Autism" at HealthImpactNews.com, February 4, 2015.

53. To read the details behind Merck's lawsuit, see "Judge: Lawsuit Against Merck's MMR Vaccine Fraud to Continue," and related articles at HealthImpactNews.com.

CHAPTER 6: LET FOOD BE THY MEDICINE

1. F. N. Jacka et al., "Maternal and Early Postnatal Nutrition and Mental Health of Offspring by Age 5 Years: A Prospective Cohort Study," *J Am Acad Child Adolesc Psychiatry* 52, no. 10 (October 2013): 1038–47, doi: 10.1016/j.jaac.2013.07.002. Also see: J. Sarris, et al., "Nutritional Medicine as Mainstream in Psychiatry," *Lancet Psychiatry* 2, no. 3 (March 2015): 271-74, doi: 10.1016/S2215-0366(14)00051-0.

2. F. N. Jacka, et al., "Does Reverse Causality Explain the Relationship between Diet and Depression?," *J Affect Disord* 175 (April 2015): 248–50, doi: 10.1016/j. jad.2015.01.007.

3. Bonnie J. Kaplan et al., "The Emerging Field of Nutritional Mental Health: Inflammation, the Microbiome, Oxidative Stress, and Mitochondrial Function." Review article for the Association for Psychological Sciences, *Clinical Psychological Science*, Sage Publications, 2014.

4. Portions of this section echo the language from my post "Enhance Your Mood with Food—Eat Naturally," www.kellybroganmd. com, October 7, 2013, http://kellybroganmd.com/article/ enhance-your-mood-with-food-eat-naturally/.

5. To read up on the work and research of Weston Price, go to his comprehensive website at www.westonaprice.org.

6. Karen Hardy et al., "The Importance of Dietary Carbohydrate in Human Evolution," *Quarterly Review of Biology* 90, no. 3 (September 2015): 251–68.

7. Stephanie Strom, "Kellogg Agrees to Alter Labeling on Kashi Line," *New York Times,* May 8, 2014, http://www.nytimes.com/2014/05/09/business/ kellogg-agrees-to-change-labeling-on-kashi-line.html.

8. The Environmental Working Group (www.ewg.org) keeps an updated list of which fruits and vegetables to buy organic. See: http://www.ewg.org/ foodnews/?gclid=Cj0KEQjwqsyxBRCIxtminsmwkMABEiQAzL34Pf-DLMtvPWcJSolmJXnLcNTlJc9P6wqTWP2VlAsJnnXIaAjIr8P8HAQ.

9. I've written extensively about glyphosate. Please visit my website for full list of citations and more information. Earth Open Source, a group of independent scientists (i.e., they are not paid to scientifically support corporations) published a compendium of literature that they called "Roundup and Birth Defects: Is the public being kept in the dark?" stating: "The pesticide industry and EU regulators knew as long ago as the 1980s to 1990s that Roundup, the world's best-selling herbicide, causes birth defects—but they failed to inform the public." The report was the by-product of an international collaboration of concerned scientists and researchers, and reveals in shocking clarity how the industry's own studies show Roundup causes birth defects in laboratory animals. Effects likely to be missed include endocrine disruption, effects on development, amplifying effects of added ingredients (adjuvants), effects of combinations of chemicals, and effects on bees. Also likely to be missed are effects found in independent peer-reviewed scientific literature, as the old directive does not explicitly say that such studies must be included in industry's dossier. In the realm of persistent and bioaccumulative pesticides and herbicides, testing only the active ingredient, or "AP," may leave manufacturers

falsely reassured. Toxicant synergy has exploded the simplistic notion of "the dose makes the poison" and a critical paper in *Biomed Research International* aimed to address flawed assumptions around pesticide and herbicide toxicity, finding that Monsanto's Roundup may be up to 10,000 times more toxic than glyphosate alone. In a 2013 paper by MIT research scientist Stephanie Seneff and an independent colleague, the effects of glyphosate on the body's microbial inhabitants were clearly described. It pointed out that among glyphosate's adverse impact, it inhibits the cytochrome P450 (CYP) enzymes, responsible for detoxifying a multitude of foreign chemical compounds, and slaughters beneficial bugs in your intestines via its impact on the "shikimate pathway" previously assumed not to exist in humans. Even vitamin D_3 activation in the liver may be negatively impacted by glyphosate's effect on liver enzymes, potentially explaining epidemic levels of deficiency.

10. K. Z. Guyton et al., "Carcinogenicity of Tetrachlorvinphos, Parathion, Malathion, Diazinon, and Glyphosate," *Lancet Oncol* 16, no. 5 (May 2015): 490–91, doi: 10.1016/S1470-2045(15)70134-8.

11. See: www.gmfreecymru.org/documents/monsanto_knew_of_glyphosate.html.

12. S. Thongprakaisang et al., "Glyphosate Induces Human Breast Cancer Cells Growth via Estrogen Receptors," *Food Chem Toxicol* 59 (September 2013): 129–36, doi: 10.1016/j.fct.2013.05.057.

13. "Egg Nutrition and Heart Disease: Eggs Aren't the Dietary Demons They're Cracked Up to Be," Harvard Health Publications, Harvard Medical School, www.health.harvard.edu/press_releases/egg-nutrition.

14. For more about the egg-cholesterol debate, see Chris Kresser's posts: "Three Eggs a Day Keep the Doctor Away," May 23, 2008, http://chriskresser.com/three-eggs-a-day-keep-the-doctor-away/, and "Why You Should Eat More (Not Less) Cholesterol," January 6, 2012, http://chriskresser.com/why-you-should-eat-more-not-less-cholesterol/.

15. C. N. Blesso et al., "Whole Egg Consumption Improves Lipoprotein Profiles and Insulin Sensitivity to a Greater Extent than Yolk-free Egg Substitute in Individuals with Metabolic Syndrome," *Metabolism* 62, no. 3 (March 2013): 400–10, doi: 10.1016/j.metabol.2012.08.014.

16. A. Vojdani and I. Tarash, "Cross-Reaction between Gliadin and Different Food and Tissue Antigens," *Food and Nutrition Sciences* 4, no. 1 (2013): 20–32, doi: 10.4236/fns.2013.41005.

17. J. Mu et al., "Interspecies Communication between Plant and Mouse Gut Host Cells through Edible Plant Derived Exosome-like Nanoparticles,"

Mol Nutr Food Res 58, no. 7 (July 2014): 1561–73, doi: 10.1002/mnfr.201300729.

18. D. L. Freed, "Do Dietary Lectins Cause Disease?" *BMJ* 318, no. 7190 (April 1999): 1023–24.

19. G. W. Tannock, "A Special Fondness for Lactobacilli," *Appl Environ Microbiol* 70, no. 6 (June 2004): 3189–94.

20. C. D'Mello et al., "Probiotics Improve Inflammation-Associated Sickness Behavior by Altering Communication between the Peripheral Immune System and the Brain," *J Neurosci* 35, no. 30 (July 29, 2015): 10821–30, doi: 10.1523/JNEUROSCI.0575-15.2015. Also see my post "Probiotics for the Brain," April 30, 2014, http://kellybroganmd.com/article/probiotics-brain/.

21. E. M. Selhub, "Fermented Foods, Microbiota, and Mental Health: Ancient Practice Meets Nutritional Psychiatry," *J Physiol Anthropol* 33 (January 15, 2014): 2, doi: 10.1186/1880-6805-33-2. Also see my post "Psychobiotics: Bacteria for Your Brain?" on GreenMedInfo.com, January 21, 2014, www.greenmedinfo.com/blog/psychobiotics-bacteria-your-brain.

22. Ghodarz Akkasheh et al., "Clinical and Metabolic Response to Probiotic Administration in Patients with Major Depressive Disorder: A Randomized, Double-blind, Placebo-controlled Trial," *Nutrition* (September 25, 2015), doi: http://dx.doi.org/10.1016/j.nut.2015.09.003.

23. A. Pärtty et al., "A Possible Link between Early Probiotic Intervention and the Risk of Neuropsychiatric Disorders Later in Childhood: A Randomized Trial," *Pediatr Res* 77, no. 6 (June 2015): 823–28, doi: 10.1038/pr.2015.51.

24. See my most at wwwkellybroganmd.com "Guts, Bugs, and Babies," August 29, 2103, http://kellybroganmd.com/article/guts-bugs-and-babies/.

CHAPTER 7: THE POWER OF MEDITATION, SLEEP, AND EXERCISE

1. The language in these paragraphs echo my post "Psychoneuroimmunology—How Inflammation Affects Your Mental Health," on April 17, 2014 at Mercola.com, http://articles.mercola.com/sites/articles/archive/2014/04/17/psychoneuroimmunology-inflammation.aspx.

2. S. W. Lazar et al., "Meditation Experience Is Associated with Increased Cortical Thickness," *Neuroreport* 16, no. 17 (November 28, 2005): 1893–97.

3. For a synthesis of the research, see Tom Ireland's blog post "What Does Mindfulness Meditation Do to Your Brain?" for *Scientific American*,

June 12, 2014, http://blogs.scientificamerican.com/guest-blog/
what-does-mindfulness-meditation-do-to-your-brain/.

4. Visit the Benson Henry Institute at www.bensonhenryinstitute.org.

5. See my well-cited article for Mercola.com "Taming the Monkey Mind—
How Meditation Affects Your Health and Wellbeing," February 20, 2014,
http://articles.mercola.com/sites/articles/archive/2014/02/20/meditation-
relaxation-response.aspx.

6. "Mindfulness Meditation Helps Fibromyalgia Patients," posted
by Brigham and Women's Hospital March 20, 2013, http://
healthhub.brighamandwomens.org/mindfulness-meditation-helps-
fibromyalgia-patients#sthash.mJ71gjem.QgviZelQ.dpbs. Also see:
Psychotherapy and Psychosomatics. "Mindfulness Meditation: A
New Treatment for Fibromyalgia?" ScienceDaily. www.sciencedaily.
com/releases/2007/08/070805134742.htm, accessed September 23,
2015. One more: E. H. Kozasa et al., "The Effects of Meditation-
based Interventions on the Treatment of Fibromyalgia," *Curr Pain
Headache Rep* 16, no. 5 (October 2012): 383–87, doi: 10.1007/
s11916-012-0285-8.

7. Michael Singer, *The Untethered Soul: The Journey Beyond Yourself* (New
York: New Harbinger, 2013). Note that the language in these paragraphs
is adapted from my post "Taming the Monkey Mind—How Meditation
Affects Your Health and Wellbeing," February 20, 2014, on Mercola.com,
http://articles.mercola.com/sites/articles/archive/2014/02/20/meditation-
relaxation-response.aspx.

8. I've written a lot about kundalini yoga online. Some of the language here
reflects my post "Kundalini Yoga: Ancient Technology for Modern Stress,"
January 6, 2014, http://kellybroganmd.com/article/kundalini-yoga/.

9. A. Goshvarpour and A. Goshvarpour, "Comparison of Higher Order
Spectra in Heart Rate Signals During Two Techniques of Meditation: Chi
and Kundalini Meditation," *Cogn Neurodyn* 7, no. 1 (February 2013): 39-
46, doi: 10.1007/s11571-012-9215-z.

10. D. Shannahoff-Khalsa, "An Introduction to Kundalini Yoga Meditation
Techniques that are Specific for the Treatment of Psychiatric Disorders,"
Journal of Alternative and Complementary Medicine 10, no. 1 (2004): 91–101.

11. L. Xie et al., "Sleep Drives Metabolite Clearance from the Adult
Brain," *Science* 342, no. 6156 (October 18, 2013): 373–77, doi: 10.1126/
science.1241224. For a full list of useful references and resources on
the power of sleep, visit the National Sleep Foundation at https://
sleepfoundation.org/.

12. P. M. Krueger and E. M. Friedman, "Sleep Duration in the United States:

a Cross-sectional Population-based Study," *Am J Epidemiol* 169, no. 9 (May 1, 2009): 1052–63, doi: 10.1093/aje/kwp023. Another great resource on sleep and the studies conducted is Dr. Michael Breus, www.thesleepdoctor. com.

13. K. Spiegel et al., "Brief Communication: Sleep Curtailment in Healthy Young Men Is Associated with Decreased Leptin Levels, Elevated Ghrelin Levels, and Increased Hunger and Appetite," *Ann Intern Med* 141, no. 11 (December 7, 2004): 846–50. Also see: University of Chicago Medical Center. "Sleep Loss Boosts Appetite, May Encourage Weight Gain." ScienceDaily. www.sciencedaily.com/releases/2004/12/041206210355.htm (accessed September 23, 2015).

14. S. Seneff, N. Swanson, and C. Li, "Aluminum and Glyphosate Can Synergistically Induce Pineal Gland Pathology: Connection to Gut Dysbiosis and Neurological Disease," *Agricultural Sciences* 6 (2015): 42–70, doi: 10.4236/as.2015.61005. Also see: J. Luke, "Fluoride Deposition in the Aged Human Pineal Gland," *Caries Res* 35, no. 2 (March-April 2001): 125–28.

15. Andrew Winokur and Nicholas Demartinis, "The Effects of Antidepressants on Sleep," *Psychiatric Times*, June 13, 2012, www. psychiatrictimes.com/sleep-disorders/effects-antidepressants-sleep.

16. Adapted from my post "Sleep: Why You Need It and How to Get It," at www.GreenMedInfo.com, August 8, 2014, www.greenmedinfo.com/ blog/sleep-why-you-need-it-and-how-get-it-2.

17. Peter L. Franzen, "Sleep Disturbances and Depression: Risk Relationships for Subsequent Depression and Therapeutic Implications," *Dialogues Clin Neurosci* 10, no. 4 (December 2008): 473–81. Also see: C. Baglioni et al., "Insomnia as a Predictor of Depression: A Meta-analytic Evaluation of Longitudinal Epidemiological Studies," *J Affect Disord* 135, no. 1–3 (December 2011): 10–9, doi: 10.1016/j.jad.2011.01.011.

18. M. Ghaly and D. Teplitz, "The Biologic Effects of Grounding the Human Body During Sleep as Measured by Cortisol Levels and Subjective Reporting of Sleep, Pain, and Stress," *J Altern Complement Med* 10, no. 5 (October 2004): 767–76.

19. Melissa Healy, "Sleeping Pills Linked to Higher Risk of Cancer, Death, Study Says," *Los Angeles Times*, February 28, 2012, http://articles.latimes. com/2012/feb/28/news/la-heb-sleep-aids-cancer-death-20120228.

20. G. S. Passos et al., "Is Exercise an Alternative Treatment for Chronic Insomnia?" *Clinics* (Sao Paulo) 67, no. 6 (2012): 653–60.

21. The volume of literature on the benefits of exercise could fill a library. You can easily check out a multitude of studies online just be googling

"benefits of exercise" or going to places like the Mayo Clinic (www. mayoclinic.org) and Harvard Health Publications (www.health.harvard. edu).

22. Dennis M. Bramble and Daniel E. Lieberman, "Endurance Running and the Evolution of *Homo*," *Nature* 432 (November 18, 2004): 345–52, doi:10.1038/nature03052.

23. A. Sierakowiak et al., "Hippocampal Morphology in a Rat Model of Depression: the Effects of Physical Activity," *Open Neuroimag J* 9 (January 30, 2015): 1–6, doi: 10.2174/1874440001509010001.

24. L. Z. Agudelo et al., "Skeletal Muscle PGC-1α1 Modulates Kynurenine Metabolism and Mediates Resilience to Stress-induced Depression," *Cell* 159, no. 1 (September 25, 2014): 33–45, doi: 10.1016/j. cell.2014.07.051. Also see: Gretchen Reynolds's coverage of this study for the *New York Times*, "How Exercise May Protect Against Depression," October 1, 2014, http://well.blogs.nytimes.com/2014/10/01/ how-exercise-may-protect-against-depression/.

25. S. Melov et al., "Resistance Exercise Reverses Aging in Human Skeletal Muscle," *PLoS One* 2, no. 5 (May 23, 2007): e465.

26. J. P. Little et al., "A Practical Model of Low-volume High-intensity Interval Training Induces Mitochondrial Biogenesis in Human Skeletal Muscle: Potential Mechanisms," *J Physiol* 588, Pt. 6 (March 15, 2010): 1011–22, doi: 10.1113/jphysiol.2009.181743.

27. G. Vincent et al., "Changes in Mitochondrial Function and Mitochondria Associated Protein Expression in Response to 2-weeks of High Intensity Interval Training," *Front Physiol* 6 (February 24, 2015): 51, doi: 10.3389/ fphys.2015.00051.

28. E. V. Menshikova et al., "Effects of Exercise on Mitochondrial Content and Function in Aging Human Skeletal Muscle," *J Gerontol A Biol Sci Med Sci* 61, no. 6 (June 2006): 534–40.

CHAPTER 8: CLEAN HOUSE

1. B. A. Cohn et al., "DDT Exposure in Utero and Breast Cancer," *J Clin Endocrinol Metab* 100, no. 8 (August 2015): 2865–72, doi: 10.1210/ jc.2015-1841.

2. You can download the bulletin here: www.acog.org/-/media/Committee- Opinions/Committee-on-Health-Care-for-Underserved-Women/ ExposuretoToxic.pdf.

3. Visit the National Institute of Environmental Health Sciences' writing on the subject matter, as well as other environmental chemicals, at www. niehs.nih.gov/health/topics/agents/endocrine/.

4. R. Yanagisawa et al., "Impaired Lipid and Glucose Homeostasis in Hexabromocyclododecane-exposed Mice Fed a High-fat Diet," *Environ Health Perspect* 122, no. 3 (March 2014): 277-83. doi: 10.1289/ehp.1307421. Also see: University of New Hampshire. "Flame retardants found to cause metabolic, liver problems, animal study shows." ScienceDaily, February 19, 2015. www.sciencedaily.com/releases/2015/02/150219101343.htm, accessed September 23, 2015.

5. Dr. Bruce Blumberg of the University of California at Irvine is credited with coining the term *obesogens*; he has spent the better part of the last decade studying the effects of chemicals on metabolism and the development of obesity—especially with regard to how risk factors for obesity due to chemical exposure can be passed on in progeny. See the following: B. Blumberg et al., "Transgenerational Inheritance of Increased Fat Depot Size, Stem Cell Reprogramming, and Hepatic Steatosis Elicited by Prenatal Exposure to the Obesogen Tributyltin in Mice," *Environ Health Perspect* 121, no. 3 (March 2013): 359-66. doi: 10.1289/ehp.1205701.

6. To read more in-depth coverage about individual chemicals and their effects, peruse the environmental medicine section of my website.

7. For facts and figures on the Body Burden, visit the Environmental Working Group at www.ewg.org.

8. Ibid.

9. Susan Freinkel, "Warning Signs: How Pesticides Harm the Young Brain," *The Nation,* March 31, 2014, www.thenation.com/article/warning-signs-how-pesticides-harm-young-brain/.

10. V. Delfosse et al., "Synergistic Activation of Human Pregnane X Receptor by Binary Cocktails of Pharmaceutical and Environmental Compounds," *Nat Commun* 6 (September 3, 2015): 8089, doi: 10.1038/ncomms9089.

11. Randall Fitzgerald, *The Hundred-Year Lie: How Food and Medicine Are Destroying Your Health* (New York: Dutton, 2006).

12. V. Delfosse et al., "Synergistic Activation of Human Pregnane X Receptor by Binary Cocktails of Pharmaceutical and Environmental Compounds," *Nat Commun* 6 (September 3, 2015): 8089, doi: 10.1038/ncomms9089.

13. Adapted from my post "Pregnant and Pre-Polluted: 8 Choices for a Healtheir Womb," July 16, 2013, http://kellybroganmd.com/article/pregnant-and-pre-polluted-8-choices-for-a-healthier-womb/.

14. R. U. Halden, "Epistemology of contaminants of emerging concern and literature meta-analysis," *J Hazard Mater* 282 (January 23, 2015): 2–9, doi: 10.1016/j.jhazmat.2014.08.074.

15. www.womensvoices.org. Also see Laura Kiesel's article for Salon, "Toxic Tampons: How Ordinary Feminine Care Products Could Be Hurting

Women," December 22, 2013, www.salon.com/2013/12/22/toxic_tampons_
how_ordinary_feminine_care_products_could_be_hurting_women/.

16. See my post "Going Organic, Down There: Feminine Products,"
November 11, 2013, http://kellybroganmd.com/snippet/going-organic-
down-there-feminine-products/. Also see: Dr. Mercola, "What's in a
Toxic Tampon," August 6, 2014, http://articles.mercola.com/sites/articles/
archive/2014/08/06/tampons-feminine-care.aspx.

17. A. M. Hormann et al., "Holding Thermal Receipt Paper and Eating Food
after Using Hand Sanitizer Results in High Serum Bioactive and Urine
Total Levels of Bisphenol A (BPA)," *PLoS One* 9, no. 10 (October 22,
2014): e110509, doi: 10.1371/journal.pone.0110509.

18. The Environmental Working Group, www.ewg.org.

19. Janet Currie et al., "Something in the Water: Contaminated Drinking
Water and Infant Health," *Canadian Journal of Economics* 46, no. 3 (August
2013): 791–810.

20. Princeton University, Woodrow Wilson School of Public and
International Affairs. "Something in the (expecting mother's) water:
Contaminated water breeds low-weight babies, sometimes born
prematurely." ScienceDaily, October 8, 2013. www.sciencedaily.com/
releases/2013/10/131008122906.htm, accessed September 28, 2015.

21. S. Roggeveen et al., "EEG Changes Due to Experimentally Induced 3G
Mobile Phone Radiation," *PLoS One* 10, no. 6 (June 8, 2015): e0129496,
doi: 10.1371/journal.pone.0129496. eCollection 2015. Also see: Sayer Ji's
article on GreedMedInfo.com, "Brain Wave Warping Effect of Mobile
Phones, Study Reveals," July 12, 2015, www.greenmedinfo.com/blog/
brain-wave-warping-effect-mobile-phones-study-reveals.

22. R. Douglas Fields, "Mind Control by Cell Phone," *Scientific American*, May
7, 2008, www.scientificamerican.com/article/mind-control-by-cell/.

23. Bin Lv et al., "The Alteration of Spontaneous Low Frequency
Oscillations Caused by Acute Electromagnetic Fields Exposure," *Clinical
Neurophysiology* 125, no. 2 (February 2014): 277–86.

24. To access Dr. Bello's list of publications, go to her site at NYU's
School of Medicine, www.med.nyu.edu/medicine/clinicalpharm/
maria-gloria-dominguez-bello-lab.

CHAPTER 9: TESTING AND SUPPLEMENTING

1. See my post "Acid Blocking Gut Sabotage," December 9, 2014, http://
kellybroganmd.com/snippet/acid-blocking-gut-sabotage/.

2. See my post "Prenatal Vitamins: A to D," April 16, 2014, http://
kellybroganmd.com/article/prenatal-vitamins-d/.

3. Patrick J. Skerrett, "Vitamin B$_{12}$ Can Be Sneaky, Harmful," Harvard Health blog, January 10, 2013, www.health.harvard.edu/blog/ vitamin-b12-deficiency-can-be-sneaky-harmful-201301105780.

4. For additional information and supporting evidence-based research on any of these supplements, visit www.kellybroganmd.com.

5. K. A. Skarupski et al., "Longitudinal Association of Vitamin B-6, Folate, and Vitamin B-12 with Depressive Symptoms among Older Adults Over Time," *Am J Clin Nutr* 92, no. 2 (August 2010): 330–35, doi: 10.3945/ ajcn.2010.29413.

6. S. Hirsch et al., "Colon Cancer in Chile Before and After the Start of the Flour Fortification Program with Folic Acid," *Eur J Gastroenterol Hepatol* 21, no. 4 (April 2009): 436–39, doi: 10.1097/ MEG.0b013e328306ccdb.

7. C. Norman Shealy et al., "The Neurochemistry of Depression," *American Journal of Pain Management* 2, no. 1 (1992): 13–16.

8. L. Sartori et al., "When Emulation Becomes Reciprocity," *Soc Cogn Affect Neurosci* 8, no. 6 (August 2013): 662–69, doi: 10.1093/scan/nss044.

9. C. M. Banki et al., "Biochemical Markers in Suicidal Patients. Investigations with Cerebrospinal Fluid Amine Metabolites and Neuroendocrine Tests," *Journal of Affective Disorders* 6 (1984): 341–50.

10. D. Benton, "Selenium Intake, Mood and Other Aspects of Psychological Functioning," *Nutr Neurosci* 5, no. 6 (December 2002): 363–74.

11. G. Shor-Posner et al., "Psychological Burden in the Era of HAART: Impact of Selenium Therapy," *Int J Psychiatry Med* 33 (2003): 55–69. Also see: L. H. Duntas et al., "Effects of a Six Month Treatment with Selenomethionine in Patients with Autoimmune Thyroiditis," *Eur J Endocrinol* 148, no. 4 (April 2003): 389–93.

12. For a summary of fish oil's effects on easing anxiety and depression, see Dr. Emily Dean's article for *Psychology Today*, "Fish Oil and Anxiety," November 10, 2011, www.psychologytoday.com/blog/ evolutionary-psychiatry/201111/fish-oil-and-anxiety.

13. www.westonaprice.org/health-topics/ cod-liver-oil-basics-and-recommendations/

14. J. Sarris et al., "S-adenosyl Methionine (SAMe) versus Escitalopram and Placebo in Major Depression RCT: Efficacy and Effects of Histamine and Carnitine as Moderators of Response," *J Affect Disord* 164 (August 2014): 76–81, doi: 10.1016/j.jad.2014.03.041.

15. V. Darbinyan et al., "Clinical Trial of Rhodiola Rosea L. Extract SHR-5 in the Treatment of Mild to Moderate Depression," *Nord J Psychiatry* 61, no. 5 (2007): 343–48.

16. A. Bystritsky et al., "A Pilot Study of Rhodiola Rosea (Rhodax) for Generalized Anxiety Disorder (GAD)," *J Altern Complement Med* 14, no. 2 (March 2008): 175–80, doi: 10.1089/acm.2007.7117.

17. S. W. Poser et al., "Spicing Up Endogenous Neural Stem Cells: Aromatic-turmerone Offers New Possibilities for Tackling Neurodegeneration," *Stem Cell Res Ther* 5, no. 6 (November 17, 2014): 127, doi: 10.1186/scrt517.

18. S. Bengmark, "Gut Microbiota, Immune Development and Function," *Pharmacol Res* 69, no. 1 (March 2013): 87–113, doi: 10.1016/j. phrs.2012.09.002. Also see my blog post "Probiotics for Prevention: The New Psychiatry," March 26, 2015, http://kellybroganmd.com/snippet/probiotics-prevention-new-psychiatry/.

19. D. Berger et al., "Efficacy of Vitex Agnus Castus L. Extract Ze 440 in Patients with Pre-menstrual Syndrome (PMS)," *Arch Gynecol Obstet* 264, no. 3 (November 2000): 150–53.

20. R. Schellenberg, "Treatment for the Premenstrual Syndrome with Agnus Castus Fruit Extract: Prospective, Randomised, Placebo Controlled Study," *BMJ* 322, no. 7279 (January 20, 2001): 134–37.

21. C. Lauritzen, "Treatment of Premenstrual Tension Syndrome with Vitex Agnus Castus Controlled, Double-blind Study versus Pyridoxine," *Phytomedicine* 4, no. 3 (September 1997): 183–89, doi: 10.1016/S0944-7113(97)80066-9.

22. J. Levine et al., "Double-blind, Controlled Trial of Inositol Treatment of Depression," *Am J Psychiatry* 152, no. 5 (May 1995): 792–94.

23. M. Fux et al., "Inositol Treatment of Obsessive-compulsive Disorder," *Am J Psychiatry* 153, no. 9 (September 1996): 1219–21.

24. V. Unfer et al., "Effects of Myo-inositol in Women with PCOS: a Systematic Review of Randomized Controlled Trials," *Gynecol Endocrinol* 28, no. 7 (July 2012): 509–15, doi: 10.3109/09513590.2011.650660.

25. V. Unfer and G. Porcaro, "Updates on the Myo-inositol Plus D-chiro-inositol Combined Therapy in Polycystic Ovary Syndrome," *Expert Rev Clin Pharmacol* 7, no. 5 (September 2014): 623-31, doi: 10.1586/17512433.2014.925795.

26. M. Gunther and K. D. Phillips, "Cranial Electrotherapy Stimulation for the Treatment of Depression," *J Psychosoc Nurs Ment Health Serv* 48, no. 11 (November 2010): 37-42. doi: 10.3928/02793695-20100701-01. 2010.

27. T. H. Barclay and R. D. Barclay, "A Clinical Trial of Cranial Electrotherapy Stimulation for Anxiety and Comorbid Depression," *J Affect Disord* 164 (August 2014): 171–77, doi: 10.1016/j.jad.2014.04.029.

CHAPTER 10: 4 WEEKS TO A NATURAL HIGH

1. S. Strauss, "Clara M. Davis and the Wisdom of Letting Children Choose Their Own Diets," *CMAJ* 175, no. 10 (November 7, 2006): 1199.
2. See "Big Pharma Hides the Truth About Coffee Enemas and Cancer," by Dr. Nicholas Gonzalez, http://thetruthaboutcancer.com/big-pharma-hides-the-truth-about-coffee-enemas-and-cancer/.
3. Michael Singer, *The Surrender Experiment* (New York: Harmony, 2015).
4. G. Chouinard and V. A. Chouinard, "New Classification of Selective Serotonin Reuptake Inhibitor Withdrawal," *Psychother Psychosom* 84, no. 2 (February 21, 2015): 63–71.
5. www.breggin.com.

CLOSING WORDS: OWN YOUR BODY AND FREE YOUR MIND

1. © The Teachings of Yogi Bhajan, circa 1977.
2. Adapted from my blog post "What Is the Point of Health?" August 4, 2015, http://kellybroganmd.com/article/whats-the-point-of-health/.
3. A. H. Maslow, "A Theory of Human Motivation," *Psychological Review* 50 (1943): 370–96.

Index

nonstick pans, 205
Nordic Cochrane Centre, 36
norepinephrine, 46, 47–48
NREM (non-rapid eye movement), 183–84
NSAIDs (non-steroidal anti-inflammatory drugs), 93–94, 128–30
nut butters, 159
nutrition. *See* diet
nuts, 159, 266
    Honey Nut Bars, 254, 289–90
    Seed Cereal, 284

obesity, 24, 88, 197, 322n5
obesogens, 197, 322n5
Occupational Safety and Health Act of 1970, 203
olanzapine, 73
omega-3 fatty acids, 162, 228
omega-6 fatty acids, 162, 228, 229
oral contraceptives, 15, 103, 115–18
organic foods, 154
Osler, William, 1
overeating, 255
oxidative stress, 117

pain management, 130
"Paleo deficit disorder," 86–87
Paleolithic diet, 28, 146–47
Pancakes, Paleo, 254, 286
pans, 205
pantothenic acid (B_5), 225
parasympathetic nervous system, 81, 172, 176, 178
Parker, William, 86
Paroxetine. *See* Paxil
pasteurization, 159
pastured animal products, 156–57
pastured eggs, 157–58
Paxil, 44, 60, 65
PBB, 195
peanuts, 159
perinatal psychiatry, 5–6
pesticides, 88, 91–92, 155–56, 200–201, 316n9
PGC-1alpha1 enzyme, 190–91
pharmaceutical industry
    data manipulation by, 44, 54
    direct-to consumer advertising and, 49, 52–55, 60
    FDA licensure requirements for, 49

    fines for fraud paid by, 138
    funding of psychiatric studies, 53
    interest in profit over professional responsibility, 5, 14, 49
    testing of antidepressants for various disorders, 42
phones, cellular, 211–13
pillows, 208
placebo effect, 54–58
plants, 208
plastic, 134, 197, 205, 208
PLOS Medicine, 49
PMS (premenstrual syndrome), 15, 116, 235
Poland, Gregory, 135
pollutants
    in municipal water, 210
    streaming of, through the placenta, 201–2
    See also chemical exposure
polyunsaturated fats, 161, 162, 228
pork
    Butternut Squash Lasagna without the Lasagna, 290–91
    Meatloaf, 254, 291–92
portion control, 142–43, 248–50
postpartum depression, 41–42, 60–61
Pottenger, Francis, 82
prebiotics, 148, 154
pregnancy
    acetaminophen during, 127
    BPA during, 133
    cesarean sections and, 84–85, 213–14
    contaminated drinking water and, 210
    exercise during, 191
    increase in psychiatric medication taken during, 42
    tapering off antidepressants when planning for, 15, 267–69
pregnenolone, 122
premenstrual syndrome (PMS), 15, 116, 235
Price, Weston A., 82, 145–46, 229
pro-inflammatory cytokines, 76
probiotics, 164–67, 234
processed foods, 148–53, 247
prolamins, 89, 103
prostaglandins, 128
proton-pump inhibitors, 93–94, 123–26
Prousky, Jonathan, 270
Prozac, 48, 52, 57, 60
psychiatric studies, funding of, 53

About the Author

KELLY BROGAN, MD, studied cognitive neuroscience at MIT before receiving her MD from Weill Cornell Medical College. Board certified in psychiatry, psychosomatic medicine, and integrative holistic medicine, she is one of the only doctors in the nation with these qualifications. She practices in Manhattan and is a mother of two young daughters.